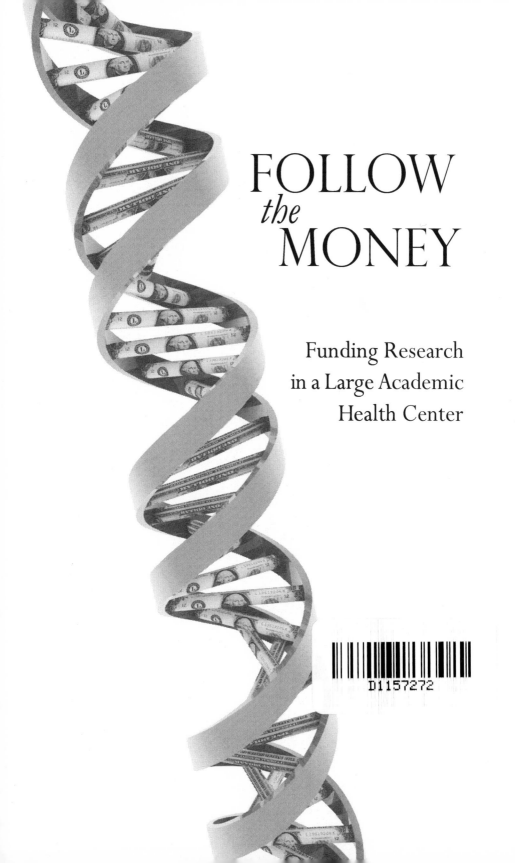

FOLLOW
the
MONEY

Funding Research
in a Large Academic
Health Center

D1157272

Perspectives in Medical Humanities

Perspectives in Medical Humanities publishes scholarship produced or reviewed under the auspices of the University of California Medical Humanities Consortium, a multi-campus collaborative of faculty, students and trainees in the humanities, medicine, and health sciences. Our series invites scholars from the humanities and health care professions to share narratives and analysis on health, healing, and the contexts of our beliefs and practices that impact biomedical inquiry.

General Editor

Brian Dolan, PhD, Professor of Social Medicine and Medical Humanities, University of California, San Francisco (UCSF)

Recent Titles

Health Citizenship: Essays in Social Medicine and Biomedical Politics
Dorothy Porter (Winter 2012)

Patient Poets: Illness from Inside Out
Marilyn Chandler McEntyre (Fall 2012) (Pedagogy in Medical Humanities series)

Bioethics and Medical Issues in Literature
Mahala Yates Stripling (Fall 2013) (Pedagogy in Medical Humanities series)

Heart Murmurs: What Patients Teach their Doctors
Edited by Sharon Dobie, MD (Fall 2014)

From Bench to Bedside, to Track & Field: The Context of Enhancement and its Ethical Relevance
Silvia Camporesi (Fall 2014)

Humanitas: Readings in the Development of the Medical Humanities
Edited by Brian Dolan (Fall 2015)

www.UCMedicalHumanitiesPress.com

brian.dolan@ucsf.edu

This series is made possible by the generous support of the Dean of the School of Medicine at UCSF, the Center for Humanities and Health Sciences at UCSF, and a University of California Research Initiative, Grant ID 141374.

Advance praise for *Follow the Money*:

This important study explores effects on an outstanding research university of a national funding crisis that threatens basic research and senior and junior biomedical researchers alike, notwithstanding large and continuing federal funding. Anyone puzzled by the contradictions facing US scientific research should read this book
—*Michael Teitelbaum*, analyst of the US scientific workforce, former Vice President of the Alfred P. Sloan Foundation, and now Senior Research Associate at Harvard's Law School.

This insightful book is a MUST read for those who serve in leadership positions in large academic health centers, or support these institutions with their strategic or financial planning.
—*Diana Carmichael*, president of AMC Strategies, a strategic planning consultant to leading US academic medical centers.

All happy institutions are alike; each unhappy institution is unhappy in its own way. Money— too little or too much, here or there—can open many possible routes to institutional unhappiness, as shown in this compelling, authoritative analysis of the finances of a leading research medical center.
—*Joseph Goldstein*, a leading investigator of cholesterol homeostasis who shared with his colleague, Michael Brown, a Lasker Award in Basic Biomedical Research, a Nobel Prize, and the National Medal of Science.

This clear account of research financing at one academic health center highlights its challenges and possible coping strategies, and exposes research funding misconceptions. It helps us understand how university based research in the US can hope to remain the envy of the world.
—*Tony Decrappeo*, President of the Council on Governmental Relations, a national association of leading research universities.

Following the financial streams of a top health sciences research institution, this book questions long-term sustainability of its research funding. An important book for any reader interested in future support of health sciences research.
—*Martha Hooven*, Vice Dean for Administration, Columbia University School of Medicine.

First published in 2016
by the University of California Medical Humanities Press
UCMedicalHumanitiesPress.com

Designed by Virtuoso Press
Cover photo courtesy of Getty Images

Library of Congress Control Number: 2016939149

ISBN: 978-0-99633242-1-2

Printed in USA

To L.H. "Holly" Smith, Jr.

Who envisioned research as the life-blood of a health

sciences university, and made it so

Contents

Acknowledgments

As beginners, we suspected this book would the first of its kind, but didn't know why. The answers were soon obvious. First, nobody else was foolhardy enough to tackle the bewildering complexities of an academic health science center. Second, people who know enough to write such a book are too busy following actual dollars in such a center to dream of writing about it. Third, such centers are rarely willing to reveal nitty-gritty details of their financial accounts, decisions, and mistakes. So, without our initial ignorance, our recent retirements from jobs at a health science center, and the generous access to key information granted by two UCSF Chancelllors, this book would not exist.

We are deeply grateful to many people who helped to repair that ignorance and make this task possible. Busy tending irons in many fires (mostly at UCSF), they gave abundant time and expertise to help us find key documents and to understand myriad rules, contradictions, policies, mistakes, and hard-won achievements. In short, they enabled us to tell a true story—despite the fact that pure and simple truth (as Oscar Wilde put it) is rarely pure and never simple.

We begin with those people who helped us understand the "big picture" at UCSF. At the outset of this project, UCSF Chancellor Susan Desmond-Hellmann gave it her blessing and correctly suggested that the two authors together could do a better job than either alone. Her successor, Chancellor Sam Hawgood, maintained his office's invaluable support and furnished useful advice and insights throughout. In addition, we are especially grateful to Dan Lowenstein, Executive Vice-Chancellor and Provost, whose thoughtful approach to problems and frank appraisals of policies, opportunities, and challenges have proved invaluable. Theresa Costantinidis, the Interim Senior Vice Chancellor – Finance & Administration, who allowed us to work closely with her staff to gather the lion's share of the data we present and discuss. Keith Yamamoto, Vice Chancellor for Policy and Strategy and Vice Dean for Research in the School of Medicine, gave us his perspective on research in basic and clinical departments.

Most UCSF staff who worked with us are long time professionals who intimately understand the institution's woof and warp. We could not have assembled the data we presented without the tireless help of Jerome Sak, Frederick Parsons and Trent Spradling, members of the UCSF Budget Office senior staff who put up with our endless questions and insatiable need to look at every tree, branch and twig in the forest. In the Budget Office, we also relied on Ann Rodriguez, Kathleen Dykhuizen-Hill, Debra Fry, Mike Clune, Bob Rhine, David Hathaway, Andrew Joseph, Chau Tu, Nilo Mia, Risa Gleichenhaus, Denis Nepveu, Taylor Mayfield, and Angie Marinello. Other UCSF administrators, analysts, and data miners who helped us in ways large and small, include John Ellis, Tammy Wallace, Shannon Turner, Lori Yamauchi, Gary Forman, Cynthia Leathers, Terri O'Brien, Jennifer O'Brien, Bob Pizzi, Steve Downs, Mike Baldelli and Mickey Zeif. We also thank Martha Hooven, currently Vice Dean of Administration at Columbia University Medical School and formerly at UCSF. Without their support this book would largely be a work of fiction.

We devoted a large fraction of our effort to exploring research and its funding in UCSF's School of Medicine. Sam Hawgood, Dean of Medicine when we began writing this book, helped to orient us before he became Chancellor. We also received excellent advice and insight from Bruce Wintroub, Chair of the Department of Dermatology, when he served as interim Dean of Medicine after Hawgood became Chancellor. We are much indebted to Talmadge King, Hawgood's successor as Dean of Medicine, for help he provided in two important roles. In his previous position, as Chair of the Department of Medicine, he had already given us invaluable information and advice. As Dean of Medicine also, we found Talmadge a fount of detailed, carefully thought-out knowledge and analysis, who communicated his comprehensive understanding in a refreshingly direct, no-nonsense way, entirely different from the friendly but sometimes blandly uninformative style affected by some high-level administrators. We also thank Maye Chrisman, in her earlier role as Associate Chair for Finance and Administration in the Department of Medicine and later in her present position as Vice Dean of Administration and Finance in the School of Medicine. Her grasp of complex details and broad understanding of the Department and the School helped us to understand both. Earlier in writing this book we also benefitted from presentations by or conversations with Mike Hindery, when he was Vice Dean for administration and finance in the School of Medicine, and Anja Paardekooper, who served as interim head of that unit between Hindery and Maye Chrisman.

We had much to learn about training young scientists at UCSF to become researchers. With respect to PhD and postdoctoral training, we received valuable orientation, advice, and data from Elizabeth Watkins, Dean of UCSF's Graduate Division and Vice Chancellor for Student Academic Affairs, and Christine Des Jarlais, Assistant Dean of the Graduate Division. Among directors of separate graduate programs, we found David Morgan, director of the UCSF Tetrad Graduate Program, especially knowledgeable and generous with his time and advice. About training young clinicians to become researchers, we learned from: Deborah Grady, who served as interim director of the Clinical and Translational Institute (CTSI) from March 2014 through January 2015; Jennifer Grandis, the present CTSI director and Associate Vice Chancellor of Clinical and Translational Research; Mike McCune and Clay Johnston, CTSI directors before Grandis; Kirsten Bibbins-Domingo; Neil Powe; William Seaman; and Mark Anderson, Director of UCSF's Medical Science Training Program. We were fortunate to get quantitative information from two experts who—among multiple other duties—made it their business to keep track on K-awardees and their training, financial support, and post-training careers: Christine Razler, Director of Research Administration in the Department of Medicine, and Christine Ireland, Deputy Director of the CTSI's Clinical and Translational Training and the K-Scholars Program.

We learned more about research in clinical departments from many faculty, chairs, and division chiefs in clinical departments, including (in addition to those noted above): Joanne Engel, Donna Ferriero, Stephen Hauser, Robert Nussbaum, Jeffrey Olgin, David Pearce, Morrie Schambelan, Kevin Shannon, Dean Sheppard, and Arthur Weiss. We also thank multiple busy K-awardees who gave us interviews about their training experience; by previous agreement, these individuals are not named here. For research in ORUs, we thank Shaun Coughlin and Jeff Bluestone. Michael Panion, a staff person in charge of finances for two clinical departments, helped us to understand research financing in those departments.

We learned about research in basic science departments from conversations with faculty members and chairs or former chairs of these departments, including: Bruce Alberts, Joe Derisi, David Julius, Brian Shoichet, Kevan Shokat, Ronald Vale, Peter Walter, and Jonathan Weissman. Susan Masters, Associate Dean of Curriculum in the School of Medicine, shared with us her earlier experience and observations when she became an adjunct faculty member charged with teaching basic science information to medical students, first primarily for in the Department of Pharmacology and later based in the Dean's Office of the School of Medicine. Mia Morgan, director of administration in the Department of Cellular and Molecular Pharmacology, helped us to understand research finances in that department.

We also learned from several individuals not directly associated with UCSF. Stephen J. Heinig, Senior Research Fellow, at the Association of American Medical Colleges, helped us to understand the AAMC's files on salaries of professors in US medical schools. Zach Hall gave us useful advice about several chapters in the book, based on his broad experience as former department chair and Vice Chancellor at UCSF, Director of the National Institute of Neurological Diseases and Stroke, and head of the California Institute for Regenerative Medicine.

Finally, we gratefully acknowledge four authorities whose writings are echoed (with many alterations) in several chapter titles. These include: Robert W. Service (chapter 3); William Shakespeare (chapters 4, 5, 7, 9); Yogi Berra (chapter 8); and James Joyce (chapter 10).

Introduction

This book seeks to explain organization and funding of biomedical research in a large academic health center, the University of California, San Francisco (UCSF). Readers of this book will learn rudiments of the finances of large academic health centers like UCSF, follow dollars in one center to understand where research money comes from and where it goes, and see how that center tries to cope with difficult challenges in the 21st century; finally, the book will weigh pros and cons of those coping strategies and suggest changes that may make some of them more effective. Most of this book's core audience, we suspect, will work at academic health centers, as researchers, physicians, teachers, leaders, administrators, students, and trainees.

Why Research? Why this book?

Why should a single US academic health center merit a book focused on its research funding? The question merits three short answers. First, for half a century, excellent research has been considered an *absolute requirement* for academic biomedical enterprises that seek to lead. We feel that research should play that essential role for the next half century and beyond, despite the many challenges this book will describe.

Second, the nation's academic health centers are complex and anomalous institutional chimeras. Few schools of any other academic discipline mix students, teachers, and researchers with a business enterprise that earns hundreds of millions of dollars every year. These health centers make crucial contributions to society and the world, but their inner workings are often mysterious to their own employees, including many researchers, teachers, and health care professionals who know little about their colleagues' work, goals, and concerns. Our bland terms for their main missions—research, education, and patient care—are much too tame to capture the internal energy, synergies, and conflicts that emit so much heat, along with dazzling flashes of light. In short, it is time for these medical centers to start understanding themselves.

Third, these large academic centers face a scary challenge: can they devise a long-term, sustainable model for funding biomedical research? The present model for delivery of clinical care works reasonably well, despite myriad glitches and problems. But in each of these centers clinical care and research exist in an uneasy tension, both competing with and depending upon one another. For such institutions—and their research—to survive, economic success of the clinical enterprise is an absolute necessity. In addition to dollars, the clinicians' focus on disease and its treatment pose critical questions, old and new, for researchers to tackle. In the opposite direction, researchers' discoveries—from the role of infectious microbes and development of antibiotics many decades ago to more recent organ transplantation, stem cells, and effective therapies for heart disease and cancer—are dramatically transforming clinical care. A once modest capacity for comforting patients and palliating symptoms has become a powerful engine for treating and preventing disease, creating an industry responsible for a large fraction of the nation's Gross Domestic Product. Every effective intervention in the clinic depends on past scientific discoveries, many of which originated in academic health centers.

In the meantime, however, it is not clear that surplus clinical income of an academic medical center can suffice to support the research mission. At present that mission depends on an unstable, cobbled-together mélange of funding from federal sources and philanthropy, plus supplements from the clinical enterprise. Can these institutions devise ways to stabilize and sustain that support over the long term?

For these three reasons, academic health centers very much merit our attention. But why, then, focus on this academic health center, UCSF? The institution does qualify as large and successful, and this book's authors both spent most of their careers at UCSF, and know it fairly well. More important, UCSF's finances are accessible to public scrutiny, because UCSF is a public institution. Accordingly, in 2013 UCSF's then Chancellor, Susan Desmond-Hellman, gave the authors permission to look into the university's books and encouraged UCSF officials to share their knowledge with us. Chancellor Sam Hawgood, her successor, did the same. For the authors this stroke of good luck was crucial, because (we suspect), no private university's health center would welcome such scrutiny. Consequently, this book's deficiencies are our own, and cannot be blamed on a secretive, uncooperative institution.

Scope and themes

The book, we hope, will challenge and intrigue its readers. Their principal challenge is the overwhelming size and complexity of the institution we describe. Indeed, writing this book repeatedly forced the authors to recognize and repair their own ignorance, despite the fact that both had spent their careers at this institution—one as a researcher and sometime department chair, the other as a financial analyst and Vice Chancellor of Finance. Similarly, chapters that bristle with complex graphs, tables, and arcana of institutional finance may daunt readers, even those familiar with a similar institution and already aware of their own ignorance. Such readers should first focus their attention on issues that affect their ability to do their jobs, skimming gory but less directly relevant complexities, to which they may return if and when the need arises.

As compensation for complexity's rigors, readers will find themselves grappling with dramatic human questions. Like the individuals whose striving lives make them work, large institutions are always driven by hope, and hope is often dashed by cold reality. Both ordinary lives and institutions run in cycles: when promise and hope fail, individuals and institutions wrestle with complication, compromise, wins, and losses. Fortunately, they usually return with renewed eagerness to tackle yet another cycle.

Like other US biomedical research centers, UCSF promises to discover new knowledge of biology, explain causes of disease, and improve its treatment. To redeem its promises, the institution confronts harsh reality in a crowded marketplace, where it weighs value and opportunity against assets, cost, and risk, and where many dollars will be gained or lost. Together, such market decisions—made by nearly 30,000 individuals, all engaged in their own promise-reality cycles—guide all UCSF's components, including its academic campus, teaching hospitals, schools, departments, laboratories, researchers, health care providers, staff, students, and faculty.

For academic biomedical researchers—including almost 2,000 faculty members at UCSF—the principal, and by far the most relentless promise-reality cycle oscillates between two poles. At one pole, the beckoning promise of biomedical science and a cornucopia of recent discoveries strongly sustain their hopes for new discoveries and miraculous disease treatments. The cornucopia's promise is real. At every level—molecules, genes, cells, the brain, the gut, the heart, the immune system, primary tumors, metastases, whole organisms, all the way to doctors and patients—hard work and modern technology can answer questions that could not even be asked ten years ago. Some of the answers, we know, will lead to profoundly useful discoveries. But the opposite pole is scary: increasingly, harsh reality discourages, delays, or prevents discovery, because dollars—grants, salaries, the cost of a critical scientific instrument—cannot be found or are already spent. A host of financial and administrative rationales, motivations, conventions, traditions, and policies—

nationally, in the government and the economy, as well as in the institution itself—intervene between an idea's promise and its realization by experiment, as this book will show.

Individual humans and large institutions resemble one another in a second way: both are driven by inherited values, learned habits, knowledge, skills, and procedures, all modified by past experience. A person's memory, learned skills, and character correspond, in institutions, nations, and businesses, to something economists call "cultural capital". Unlike revenues, expenses, costs, loans, assets, liabilities, risks, margins, losses, capital expenditures, and ordinary economic capital, cultural capital is hard to quantify, but can generate immense power—as Aztecs learned from Cortez, and climate scientists find when they try to persuade us to reduce our reliance on fossil fuels.

Every quantifiable variable at UCSF—and every dollar from any source that goes to this or that destination—depends directly on the state of at least one fierce (but often quiet) struggle waged between distinct human "cultures." These cultures may belong to different institutions—another university, a competing deliverer of patient care, a government agency, or the US Congress—or, within UCSF, to specific missions, including research, teaching, patient care, and their many sub-varieties. Each such culture—readers will encounter at least one on almost every page of this book—has its own leaders, followers, bedrock tenets, traditions, convictions, unifying drives and sub-divisions, virtues and faults. Over time each culture competes against or synergizes with others, changes in myriad ways, may subdivide itself, and (eventually) dies.

How to use this book

Science inevitably produces change. That is how the triumphs of 20th-century biomedical research unleashed external forces that push the biomedical science culture toward further changes today. External pressures do not always point in the right direction, however. Can the biomedical research culture grasp its own destiny by deliberately choosing which paths to take? Or will it avoid such choices until external change steers it in directions it cannot tolerate? The answers depend on how well the research culture understands its environment and its own workings. A few senior scientists urged one of the authors not to write this book, because it might discourage young people from embarking on research careers and demoralize striving young scientists. Their *sotto voce* argument: only the old guard can be trusted to handle sordid money questions. The argument is wrong, for closely related reasons:

1. Young scientists and would-be scientists *must* learn about money, because their futures critically depend on it, and because they will soon be in charge.
2. The immense promise of 21st-century research can be realized only if institutions and researchers learn how to spend their money, and when not to spend it.
3. No scientist, leader of science, or reader can afford to ignore the powerful leverage furnished by understanding any complex mechanism—how bases pair in a double helix, how AIDS viruses replicate, or how large institutions finance research.

Because scientists who understand science funding can do better science, this book can be useful in three different ways. First, it serves as a primer and guide for students, professors, staff, administrators, and academic leaders who need to navigate the maze of revenues, expenses, governance, and academic cultures that controls biomedical research within large US research universities. The primer focuses on one such university, but will prove a useful guide to parallel complexities in many, because underlying themes vary little, even when details differ. Second, some facts and inferences in this book will furnish genuine surprises for readers who explore mysteries of indirect cost recovery, faculty researcher salaries paid from sponsored projects, endowments, capital investments, or different research cultures. The surprises will educate naïve beginners, while veterans who venture beyond their own well-tended gardens will discover flora and fauna in many a neighboring wilderness.

In addition to serving as a guide through complexity and a vehicle for education and surprise, we hope this book's inferences and interpretations, hard questions and tentative answers will persuade readers to think hard about how to sustain the fragile ecosystem of academic biomedical research for the next 10, 20, or 50 years. While the book's quantitative facts are as accurate as we could make them, our inferences or interpretations deal with ever-shifting human attitudes and behaviors, where categorical black and white judgments can be right, wrong, or sometimes both at once. We urge readers to tackle our questions, interpretations, and proposed remedies head-on, instead of dismissing them outright as simply wrong, or perhaps right but irrelevant to their own particular situation. Some of this book's questions may be poorly framed, its interpretations mistaken, and its proposals inadequate. But close examination will reveal the extreme fragility of academic biomedical research, and—we believe—the root cause of that fragility: that curiosity-driven research can never thrive under conditions that require it to produce profit or even to support itself, over the short term; instead, its real long-term value—medical, social, or economic—absolutely *requires* it to fail more often than it succeeds. In a "business model" society driven by short-term rewards, research's long-term rewards require long-term investments. Readers who confront this paradox head on can ask better questions, provide more correct interpretations, and—if we are lucky—craft corrective actions that work.

Finally, the rest of this book is organized in 10 chapters, which begin by sketching UCSF as a research university, and then proceed through its complex human and financial components. Chapter 1 first presents the financial "big picture" of UCSF as it was in Fiscal Year 2014 (FY2014), as well as its remarkable expansion and increases in revenue over the past 30 years, and then sketches changes within and outside the university that pose major challenges. Chapters 2-6 explore: revenue streams; investments, endowments, and research facilities; indirect costs of research (i.e., dollars not paid by grants to investigators); how decisions are made to distribute research money, hire faculty, and start new projects; and how patient care revenues, research grants, and university coffers support faculty salaries and benefits. Interpretations and inferences abound in chapters 7-9, which focus on the organization and funding of research and graduate education in basic science and clinical departments, as well as the fertile and sometimes conflicted relations between clinical and "basic" research. In chapters 1-9, the primary aim is to describe, analyze, diagnose, and identify major issues—that is, not to prescribe remedies but to provide information that may enable readers to devise their own remedies. The final chapter summarizes UCSF's present successes, many challenges it faces, and dangerous threats to sustaining its research mission. Then it proposes changes that may allow UCSF and other research universities to handle both their successes and their challenges more effectively.

Chapter 1

Today's enterprise reflects decades of change

The University of California, San Francisco (UCSF) comprises a health care system and four Schools—Dentistry, Nursing, Pharmacy, and Medicine. In multiple hospitals and two main academic campuses, it pursues three missions: education, research, and treatment of disease. In fiscal year 2014 (FY2014), UCSF employed 22,928 people, and earned revenues of $4.45 billion (B) per year (1). It taught 5,632 students and trainees (that is, graduate professional students, graduate PhD and MS students, postdocs, and residents; 1). Its hospitals admitted 29,230 patients and managed 963,692 outpatient visits (2). In the same fiscal year, it received $992 million (M) in federal, state and private grants or contracts designated to support research (3). Together, these research dollars accounted for 22% of UCSF's total revenues, and a much larger proportion (48%) of those of its academic core, or Campus, as distinguished from (and not including) its clinical enterprise. In size and quality, UCSF's clinical care and research both rank consistently among the top US academic medical centers.

As the 21st century unfolds, UCSF takes pride in its accomplishments and delight in its future prospects. Still, dark clouds loom, all related to problems UCSF shares with other leading US academic biomedical centers. First, UCSF's size and multifarious missions make it so complex that many faculty—and even some officials and financial gurus—do not understand how it works. Many faculty and employees remain confused about where UCSF gets its money and how it is spent. UCSF's diverse missions complement and reinforce, but also compete against and hinder one another. Not knowing where the dollars flow makes it harder for proponents of each separate mission to assess their roles and contributions in relation to those of their competitors.

Second, unpredictable economic, social, and political changes threaten the fiscal integrity of UCSF and other biomedical research institutions: the US economy is still recovering from a major recession; federal and state governments become less and less willing to increase or even stably maintain financial support for clinical care, research, and education; costs of faculty and employee salaries, health benefits, and pensions continue to rise; as patient populations age and need complex new therapies, costs of clinical care dramatically increase; modes of payment for clinical care appear increasingly volatile and unstable; driven by opportunities for improving human welfare, biomedical research expands and becomes even more expensive.

Finally, in addition to external threats, UCSF—again, like many other academic medical centers—faces crucial internal dilemmas created by its own success. These affect all UCSF's missions, but none more profoundly than its research. UCSF's research mission, the primary focus of this and subsequent chapters, requires the institution to grapple with internal dilemmas that involve governance, long-standing programs, salaries, other financial commitments, choices among competing scientific questions, and different goals for the rate and direction of the institution's growth and the quality of its research. Failure to understand how the institutional "machine" works can delay or distort crucial decisions and recognition of hidden problems, some of which may require UCSF to revise or even discard inherited habits and practices.

The potential dangers of misunderstanding prompted this book's focus on financing research at UCSF. We shall "follow the money" as it flows into UCSF's biomedical research, within the larger context of an institution that also pursues critical missions in education and patient care. In following research dollars, we shall often treat other missions as detail-free "black boxes," except in cases where either mission impinges directly on research—e.g., in teaching PhD student researchers or in using patient care revenues to support research.

To set the stage for describing specific aspects of UCSF's research finances, this first chapter presents the current "big picture" snapshot of UCSF and sketches dramatic changes over three decades that created major challenges. Remarkably, these challenges prevented neither continuing expansion of UCSF's revenues nor the growing strength of its missions, including research. Such success, in the face of profound change, attests to the extraordinary ingenuity, ability, and motivation of UCSF's people, who constitute the bulk of its collective "cultural capital," as we indicated in the Introduction. It is also worth emphasizing that UCSF is one of many US research institutions that face the same difficult challenges and profound changes in the 21st century, as indicated in broad overviews of the finances of such institutions (4,5).

Governance

As a center for health science education, research, and clinical care, UCSF is one of the ten campuses of the University of California (UC). Fig. 1-1a shows UCSF's formal governance, including executives who make high-level executive decisions. At the top is the Chancellor (Sam Hawgood, appointed by UC's President in July 2014). As chief administrative officer, the Chancellor presides over both UCSF's Campus, or academic core, and its clinical enterprise, which was termed the Medical Center (MC) until July 2014, when it became UCSF Health. The Chancellor appoints the Chief Executive Officer (CEO)

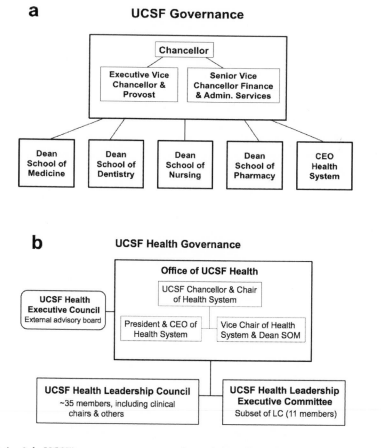

Fig. 1-1 a & b. UCSF's governance structure. See main text for explanation of the governance of UCSF (panel a) and UCSF Health (panel b). Abbreviations: Administration; CEO, chief executive officer; LC, Leadership Council; SOM, School of Medicine.

of UCSF Health, deans of the Schools of Dentistry, Nursing, Pharmacy, and Medicine, and vice chancellors in charge of various administrative activities within the Chancellor's office. Deans administer education and research in their Schools through the chairpersons of academic departments.

The Office of UCSF Health (Fig. 1-1b) comprises the Chancellor and two of his appointees: Mark Laret, President and CEO of the UCSF Health System, and the Dean of the School of Medicine, Talmadge King, is also vice chair of UCSF Health. (The Chancellor appointed King, formerly chair of the medical school's Department of Medicine, to the deanship in May, 2015.) The Office of UCSF Health administers the clinical enterprise through a "board" or Leadership Council (health system executives and chairs of clinical departments in the School of Medicine), plus other committees (not in the Figure) composed of clinical department chairs and faculty members.

Governance charts tend to mask troublesome devils-behind-the-details, many of which we'll meet in later chapters. Here we sketch three of the most important:

1. *UCSF's missions overlap and compete* for space, money, and faculty time and effort.
2. *Who is in charge?* Governance charts formally depict which administrator reports to which superior official, but not the real distribution of power, which at UCSF is especially strong at the levels of clinical specialties in UCSF Health and of Campus departments, relative to deans of Schools and the Chancellor's office.
3. *Size differences among entities within administrative units.* The clinical enterprise brings in 54% of UCSF's total income (Fig. 1-2a; 1), including professional fees that pay many faculty; the School of Medicine accounts for 86% of Campus expenditures attributable to Schools (6); within the School of Medicine, the Department of Medicine earns and spends more than 20% of all revenues—more, indeed, than the combined revenues and expenses of 24 of the School's 43 departments (6); several of that Department's subspecialty divisions are bigger and more complex than many academic departments.

All major academic health centers face similar hidden devils, with variations that reflect separate evolutionary paths and environments. As such enterprises grow, inevitable internal tensions among diverse goals, levels of power, and different-sized functional units can threaten to make old challenges worse and to slow or inhibit nimble responses to unpredictable new challenges from the

Total Revenues (FY2014): $4.45B

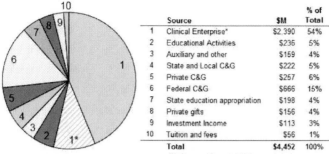

	Source	$M	% of Total
1	Clinical Enterprise*	$2,390	54%
2	Educational Activities	$236	5%
3	Auxiliary and other	$159	4%
4	State and Local C&G	$222	5%
5	Private C&G	$257	6%
6	Federal C&G	$666	15%
7	State education appropriation	$198	4%
8	Private gifts	$156	4%
9	Investment Income	$113	3%
10	Tuition and fees	$56	1%
	Total	**$4,452**	**100%**

Professional fees of $449M are included

Fig. 1-2a

Campus Revenues (FY2014): $2.06B

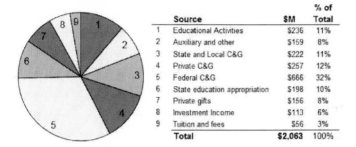

	Source	$M	% of Total
1	Educational Activities	$236	11%
2	Auxiliary and other	$159	8%
3	State and Local C&G	$222	11%
4	Private C&G	$257	12%
5	Federal C&G	$666	32%
6	State education appropriation	$198	10%
7	Private gifts	$156	8%
8	Investment Income	$113	6%
9	Tuition and fees	$56	3%
	Total	**$2,063**	**100%**

Fig. 1-2b

Fig. 1-2. Revenues in FY2014. Panels present revenue streams of: (a) all of UCSF, including the clinical enterprise; (b) the Campus only, excluding the clinical enterprise. Data derived from reference 1 and 3. The table lists each revenue stream with a number (from 1-10) that corresponds to numbers of the pie slices in panel a or the nine slices in panel b, in clockwise order (except that number 10, the extremely thin tuition and fees slice, is not numbered in the pie diagram of panel a). Close inspection reveals that three revenue categories here differ from those depicted in the temporal trends shown in Figs. 4 and 5 (see also, Fig. 4 legend). The most striking is the Professional Fees category ($449M) (7), which is marked with an asterisk (1*) and cross-hatched in panel a. These funds are formally part of the Clinical Enterprise, and are simply included in that larger category in the graphs of trends from FY1984 to FY2014. In FY2014 and previous years UCSF always included professional fees as revenue of the clinical enterprise, because they were largely collected by the teaching hospitals. After collection, these funds are transferred to the Campus, which distributes them to academic clinical departments that pay salaries to faculty engaged in patient care. Two other changes resulted in appearance of new categories (shown in panels a and b) that are not separately depicted in Figs. 1-4 and 1-5: private gifts (no. 8 in Fig. 2-2a) are included in the private gifts, contracts and grants category of Figs. 1-4 and 1-5; investment income (no. 9 in Fig. 1-2) was included in the "auxiliary and other" category of Figs. 1-4 and 1-5.

outside. These chapters focus on challenges that affect UCSF's research and how UCSF responds to them.

Revenues and expenditures

To help keep our bearings as we explore the complex maze of UCSF's research finances, we begin with low-resolution snapshots of the institution's financial landscape in FY2014 (*1*). Significant proportions of UCSF's total $4.452B in revenues in that year (Fig. 1-2a) include federal, state and private contracts and grants (together, 27%, primarily for research), professional fees (10%) (*7*), and patient care revenues of UCSF's clinical enterprise (44%). No other revenue category brings in more than 5% of the total.

Relative sizes of academic revenues stand out more prominently if we depict them as proportions of the academic Campus by itself (that is, the "academic" 46% that remains after excluding the clinical enterprise; Fig. 1-2b). The largest slices of this $2.062B Campus pie are: federal contracts and grants (32% of Campus revenues); private contracts and grants (12%); state and local contracts and grants (11%); a grab-bag category vaguely termed "educational activities" (11%), which represents a miscellany of sales and services related to clinical care, along with a few genuinely educational activities; and educational appropriations from the state of California (10%). Four remaining categories (private gifts, auxiliary and other, investment income, and student tuition and fees) together account for ~24% of Campus revenues.

In FY2014 the largest expenditures (Fig. 1-3) of both the Campus (67%) and the clinical enterprise (61%) went to employee salaries and benefits, such as the employer's share of pension funds, health insurance, etc. Expenses of the clinical enterprise for materials, supplies, and utilities (33%) proportionately exceed those of the Campus (25%).

This low-resolution view reveals two important sets of facts: (i) the clinical enterprise accounts for a large proportion of UCSF's revenues, and allows clinical faculty to earn professional fees that pay substantial proportions of their salaries; (ii) most Campus revenues depend on federal and private contracts and grants for research, plus professional fees brought in by faculty clinicians, with smaller amounts from the state (for teaching) or from auxiliary sales and services. In subsequent essays we shall see how these facts influence UCSF's priorities and research goals.

Clinical Enterprise Expenses (FY2014): $1.79B

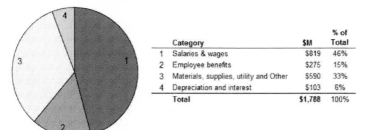

	Category	$M	% of Total
1	Salaries & wages	$819	46%
2	Employee benefits	$275	15%
3	Materials, supplies, utility and Other	$590	33%
4	Depreciation and interest	$103	6%
	Total	$1,788	100%

Fig. 1-3a

Campus Expenses (FY2014): $2.50B

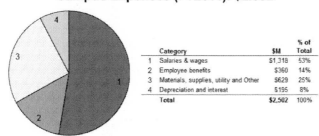

	Category	$M	% of Total
1	Salaries & wages	$1,318	53%
2	Employee benefits	$360	14%
3	Materials, supplies, utility and Other	$629	25%
4	Depreciation and interest	$195	8%
	Total	$2,502	100%

Fig. 1-3b

Fig. 1-3. Expenses in FY2014. Panels present expenditures of: (a) the clinical enterprise; (b) the Campus only, excluding the clinical enterprise. Data derived from reference *1*. As in Fig. 1-2, in each panel each numbered expense category (in the table) corresponds to a pie slice (numbered in clockwise order).

Growth over three decades

To capture trends and striking changes in UCSF's finances over the past three decades, we plot UCSF's revenues from FY1984 through FY2013 (*8*). The resulting graphs present these revenues in various accounting categories—that is, the Campus plus the clinical enterprise (here termed Teaching Hospitals) (Fig. 1-4) or Campus revenues only (Fig. 1-5, excluding Teaching Hospitals). Both figures present the categories on three different scales: nominal US dollars (panels 1-4a or 1-5a); 1984 dollars, thus correcting subsequent values for inflation (panels 1-4b or 1-5b) (*9*); or as a percentage of the whole UCSF or Campus budget for that year (panels 1-4c or 1-5c). (Two small points, related to accounting changes: (i) revenue categories in FY2013 and previous years differ slightly from those of FY2014, as described in the legends of Figs. 1-2 and 1-4; (ii) boxes at the center of all panels of Figs. 1-4 and 1-5 obscure data from FY1998-2000, because transient changes in accounting practices during those years, related to the temporary merger of UCSF's MC with Stanford Health Services, produced distracting aberrations that are not relevant to our conclusions and inferences.

Fig. 1-4 shouts one message, loud and clear: revenue growth of UCSF's medical teaching hospitals dwarfs changes in all other categories. Over three decades the teaching hospitals (dark blue, in each panel) grew 17.7-fold from $135M to $2.39B, in nominal US $ (Fig. 1-4a). Even corrected for inflation (Fig. 1-4b), over this 30 years Teaching Hospital revenue grew to 5.9-fold its size in FY1984, while combined (and inflation-corrected) Campus revenue barely doubled (2.1-fold). Overall, in 1984 dollars, UCSF's revenues increased to 3.4-fold its size 30 years earlier. In 1984 dollars, of the $1.073B increase in all revenues, the clinical enterprise accounted for $681M, or 64%. Consequently, by FY2014 the Teaching Hospitals accounted for 54% of UCSF's total revenues, or ~1.8-fold its percentage in FY1984; conversely, the academic Campus's share decreased from 70% to 46% (Fig. 1-4c).

Data in Fig. 1-4 support two inferences. First, the clinical enterprise's remarkable growth reflects its high standards for delivering clinical care and skills and hard work of staff and leadership in a tough competitive environment. Indeed, the inflation-corrected 5.9-fold change in Teaching Hospital revenues over three decades (Fig. 1-4b) exceeds the approximate quintupling (*10*) of overall US healthcare spending (also inflation-corrected) during the same period. Second, it is likely that the growing financial predominance of clinical

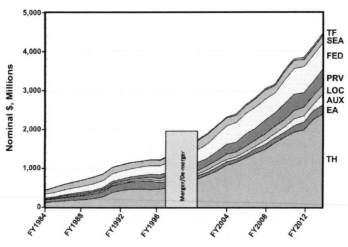

Fig. 1-4a

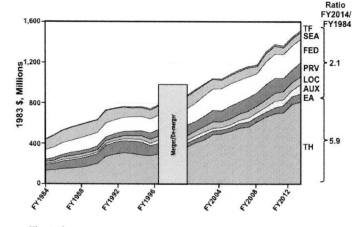

Fig. 1-4b

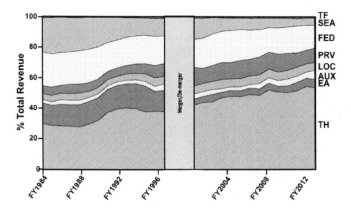

Fig. 1-4c

Fig. 1-4. Trends of UCSF's revenue streams, including both the Campus and the clinical enterprise, over three decades, from FY1984 to FY 2014 (8). Panels present separate revenue streams: (a) in nominal dollars; (b) in inflation-corrected 1984 dollars (9); (c) as percentages of UCSF's total revenues for each fiscal year. Revenue categories are identical in all 3 panels, arranged in order (top to bottom of each graph): student tuition and fees (TF); state educational appropriation (SEA); federal contracts and grants (Fed); private C&G and gifts (PRV); Local and state C&G (LOC); Auxiliary and other (AUX); educational activities (EA); Teaching Hospitals (TH, aka the clinical enterprise). Vertical boxes, marked Merger/De-merger, obscure misleading, bumpy data from years in which the clinical enterprises of UCSF and Stanford University transiently merged, then de-merged (see main text); in this regard, note that dollars assigned to the EA category are conspicuously lower after than before the merger/demerger, a change that largely reflects transfer of professional fees from EA to the teaching hospital, and thus contribute to (but do not fully account for) the large and persistently increasing apparent growth of the clinical enterprise. Note that the detailed breakdown of revenue categories differs slightly from those in Fig. 1-2, as explained in the Fig. 1-2 legend.

care, in comparison to academic research and teaching, has exerted significant effects on UCSF's values, governance, and development, and must have also garnered greater attention and effort from institutional leaders. More directly relevant to our main concern with research, growth in clinical care revenues requires more faculty physicians, many of whom also become researchers in clinical departments—and seek more grant money, laboratory space and facilities, students, postdocs, and technicians.

Fig. 1-4c depicts the various revenue categories as percentages of total UCSF revenues over the years: strikingly, the proportionately large relative growth of UCSF's clinical enterprise was accompanied by an equally impressive proportional dwindling of state appropriations to UCSF for education. As we shall see, the opposite changes in these two revenue categories, state funds and clinical enterprise revenues, pose important challenges for UCSF in the 21st century.

Trends in Campus revenues over the past three decades (Fig. 1-5) highlight both the decrease in state support for education and impressive increases in research support. A quick glance at Campus revenue trends in nominal US dollars (Fig. 1-5a) may suggest that revenue categories increased in roughly the same proportion, but that impression is wrong. For instance, correcting revenues in these categories for inflation (Fig. 1-5b) shows clearly that state educational appropriations *decreased* by ~30% from FY1984 to FY2014, while overall Campus revenues increased 2.3-fold. Now, as in the past, those state funds primarily support faculty salaries, and more especially those of researchers who cannot earn professional fees for patient care. In contrast, revenue categories primarily related to research increased markedly: by FY 2014, fed-

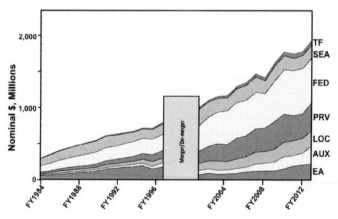

Fig. 1-5a

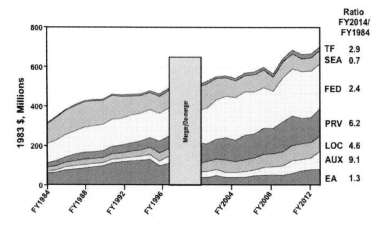

Fig. 1-5b

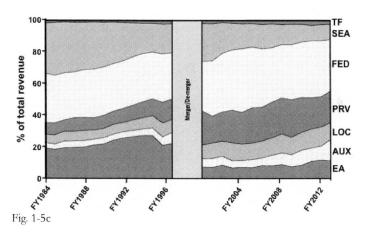

Fig. 1-5c

Fig. 1-5. Trends of the revenue streams of UCSF's Campus, excluding the clinical enterprise, over three decades, from FY1984 to FY 2014 (8). Panels present separate revenue streams: (a) in nominal dollars; (b) in inflation-corrected 1984 dollars (9); (c) as percentages of UCSF's total revenues for each fiscal year. Abbreviations of revenue sources are as specified in the legend of Fig. 1-4. For vertical boxes, marked Merger-Demerger, see legend to Fig. 1-4. The revenue categories shown differ from those in Fig. 1-2, as explained in the Fig. 1-2 legend.

eral contracts brought in 2.4-fold greater revenues than in FY1984; for private gifts, grants & contracts the increase was much larger, to 6.2-fold. By FY2014, these two categories, which predominantly pay for research, together accounted for 24% of total UCSF revenues (Fig. 1-4a) and 52% of Campus revenues (Fig. 1-5a). Corrected for inflation, FY2014 revenues from local and state contracts, which relate primarily to clinical services, increased 4.6-fold over three decades, and the Auxiliary and other category (which includes largely self-supporting services like parking and housing) grew 9.1-fold. Student tuition and fees (from matriculated professional and graduate students) grew 2.9-fold, but still account for a tiny fraction of UCSF's revenues.

Finally, considering these revenue categories as percentages of all Campus revenues (Fig. 1-5c) draws the starkest picture. In the early 1980s, as an academic Campus UCSF derived about one third of its revenues in the form of tax-derived dollars from the state of California, predominantly in the form of salaries for its faculty (that is, state educational appropriations). By 2014 the faculty had grown much larger, but tax-supported faculty salary support from the university had decreased 3-fold, to barely 10% of Campus revenues. Where did UCSF's faculty find salary money to replace the missing state appropriations? By and large, clinicians derived ever-greater proportions of their salary from delivery of health care services. Lacking that option, most PhD researchers had to garner more salary from research-targeted contracts, grants, and gifts to them and the Campus. For decades, federal plus private support for research have constituted a substantial fraction of UCSF's Campus revenues: that fraction grew from ~39% in the early 1980s to ~52% in FY2014. Although UCSF remains a leading target for federal research support (~31% vs. 32% of Campus revenues in FY1984 vs. FY2014), the private sector (predominantly industry) accounted for 21% of Campus revenues in FY2014, vs. 7% in FY1984.

In summary, the low-resolution picture of financial trends in Figs. 4 and 5 reveals key features of UCSF's past and present, and suggests auguries for its future.

1. In the early 1980s, the institution's effort, apportioned almost equally between medical care delivery and biomedical research, was held together by generous support for its Campus by taxpayers, through the University of California.
2. Subsequent rapid growth of its clinical activities, in combination with curtailed taxpayer contributions to academic missions, converted UCSF into a predominantly clinical enterprise with a substantial research component and a faculty whose salaries depend increasingly on clinical work and/or grant dollars.
3. Increasing predominance of the health-care mission bolsters the research mission by attracting clinically competent faculty who also engage in research. At the same time, their clinically oriented research competes for institutional attention and resources against more basic research.

4. At present the clinical enterprise's prosperity and momentum help to support all of UCSF, but health care's large share of US GDP (almost double that of many other developed countries; *11*) may not always be sustained. Should UCSF diversify its part of the health-care juggernaut and curb its headlong growth?

5. UCSF's research—clinical, basic, and in between—remains vibrant and productive, but risks outgrowing available funding, especially from the federal government.

Future challenges

This chapter has sketched UCSF's governance structure, outlined its current revenues and expenses, and revealed major changes in its revenue pattern over the past three decades. To conclude, here we summarize major financial and other challenges that are highlighted in subsequent chapters, under three general headings.

Changes outside UCSF underlie many present challenges, including:

1. Ever-decreasing availability of state funds, as taxpayers become less willing to continue paying for education and research.

2. Decreases in previously generous support from the federal government for education, patient care, and—just as crucially—biomedical research.

3. A major economic recession, now slowly resolving, sapped political support for governmental investment in academic research, education, and patient care, and also damped private giving and support for collaborative research from industry.

4. The highly competitive health care industry has rapidly expanded, but also fears potential instabilities produced by controversy over government support for medical care and rising costs and complexity of drugs and other therapies.

5. In the US and internationally, both basic and applied biomedical research are subject to rapid change and strong competition.

Reduced available resources, imbalanced missions, and increasing costs of doing business all reflect effects of external changes beyond control of UCSF, including:

6. Loss of state revenues forces UCSF's missions to compete against one another, leading clinicians to suspect that a portion of their professional fees is distributed disproportionately to support education and research,

and researchers and educators to worry that UCSF does not sufficiently value their contributions.

7. Driven by inflation and competitive hiring by other institutions, faculty and staff salaries and benefits (e.g., pensions and medical insurance) continue to rise, reducing funds available for programmatic and strategic purposes.

8. Employee pensions since 1990 required no UCSF contributions, but owing to the recent economic recession in FY2012 UCSF was required in to support pension funds with dollars that added 8% to its total salary expenditures; now this extra contribution from UCSF's coffers has risen to 14% of salary expenditures (*12*).

Intrinsic characteristics and practices reduce institutional flexibility and responsiveness to new challenges:

9. Creaky, bottom-up traditions of campus governance change slowly and tightly constrain responses to rapid changes in UCSF's environment.

10. Rapid expansion of both research laboratories and clinical facilities imposes large debt obligations. By FY2025, planned construction and renovation are projected to double the cost of servicing debts (interest), to ~$231M per year (*13,14*), making it harder to fund strategies for tackling new challenges while maintaining existing programs and facilities.

11. External funds, federal and private, pay very large fractions of many researchers' salaries, putting hundreds of faculty at risk if external sources diminish further and impairing mutual loyalties of UCSF and its research faculty to each other.

12. Despite evidence that available resources are limited, UCSF as a whole behaves as if quality and quantity are synonyms, and exhibits little interest in plans that do not require expansion of personnel, facilities, and programs. Should UCSF try more actively to shape new directions for its research and clinical juggernauts, or hang on and enjoy both rides while they last?

Our chapters will repeatedly encounter each of these challenges. Their resemblance—financial (*4*) and otherwise—to challenges faced by other academic research centers should strike responsive chords in scientists, physicians, students, administrators, staff, and patients whose lives and hopes depend on the future of academic biomedical research.

Chapter 2

Revenue generates and constrains opportunity

Academic research institutions constantly weigh tempting opportunities against limited and constrained resources. Opportunities always cost money, ranging from the relatively small ($~0.5-2.0M) start-up fund for a hot-shot young researcher, to several $M for an academic program focused on a new field, to more than $1B for constructing, equipping, and populating the first buildings of a new campus. For UCSF, a $4.452B-per-year enterprise, potential resources for pursuing such opportunities fall under three headings: (i) Relatively reliable revenue streams from many sources; (ii) gifts and endowments; (iii) physical space and facilities, produced by capital investment of philanthropic gifts and loans. This chapter, along with chapters 3, 4, and 5, will explain these financial resources, constraints and opportunities associated with each, and how UCSF uses its "margin" between revenue and expense. ("Margin," the institutional term for what an ordinary business calls profit, provides financial elbow-room for achieving future aspirations.) This background information will set the stage for exploring UCSF's research finances in detail. The present chapter focuses on reliable revenue streams and gifts and endowments.

Revenue streams

These "streams" derive from UCSF's ongoing operations, in amounts that change relatively little from year to year but can trend substantially upward or downward over longer periods. Concentrating primarily on FY2014 revenues, we describe in more detail the revenue streams introduced in chapter 1, and indicate whether and to what degree UCSF can use each category's revenue to tackle new opportunities.

Clinical revenues. Six-fold growth over 30 years made UCSF's teaching hospitals the institution's largest single revenue generator ($2.39B, or 54% of its total revenues in FY2014; *1*). UCSF currently operates hospitals on three separate campuses in San Francisco (Parnassus, Mt. Zion, and Mission Bay), plus another across the Bay, the Benioff and Oakland Children's Hospital. In addition, UCSF assists the City and County of San Francisco in operating San Francisco General Medical Center and provides operational support to the Ft. Miley VA Medical Center in San Francisco. Each hospital serves as a training site for UCSF medical, nursing and pharmacy students. The hospitals also allow UCSF physicians to generate professional fee income ($449M; 2), collected by the clinical enterprise and transferred to the Campus. Professional fees still counted as Medical Center revenue for FY2014, but in reality, this revenue category "belongs" to both segments of the UCSF enterprise (see below).

Grants and contracts for research. This revenue source pumps most of the blood that sustains UCSF's research and teaching missions. In FY2014, it came to $992M and accounted for 55% of Campus revenues or 26% of total UCSF revenues (1). "Sponsored" research grants and contracts are formal agreements with external sponsoring parties in which UCSF promises to provide specific outcomes that meet those parties' needs for research to create new knowledge. Most sponsored research funds ($665M, which includes $152M in indirect costs, as described later) come from federal sources like the National Institutes of Health (NIH) and the National Science Foundation, plus smaller contributions from the Departments of Education, Energy, and Defense. In addition, sponsored research agreements with non-federal funders (1, 3) come from two kinds of sources. (i) philanthropic foundations (e.g., American Heart Association, American Cancer Society, Juvenile Diabetes Foundation) seeking to understand and treat human diseases ($190M); or (ii) pharmaceutical companies which wish to develop or test the performance of a new therapy in trials with patients suffering from a particular disorder ($22M). Total revenues for non-federally sponsored research in FY2014 come to $257M, including indirect costs of $45M (4). In addition, the state of California provides $66M to UCSF to conduct research; most of this money comes from either the California Institute for Regeneration Medicine or from federal funds that flow through state agencies to UCSF; of this $66M, less than $9M is for indirect costs (4).

Most of the funds in sponsored research agreements, called "direct costs," pay salaries and benefits of faculty who direct the research and postdoctoral scholars and technicians who conduct it in the laboratory, as well as research supplies, materials, and equipment; they can also support tuition and salary stipends for graduate students working on funded projects. Flowing through the UCSF Campus to researchers, these costs contribute directly to producing new knowledge. Direct costs cannot be used for purposes separate from the specific research described in the sponsored agreement, however, not even to pay incurred (but "indirect") costs that relate to and are necessary for the research to be performed, such as electricity, heating, lab construction or renovation, administrative support, and certain other expenses. In FY2014 UCSF recovered $197M in indirect costs (7.9% of Campus revenue; *4*). While recovery of indirect costs is governed by an immense set of arcane rules and procedures (for more detail, see chapter 3), it provides a somewhat flexible, but still highly constrained, source of funds for research opportunities (see chapter 5).

Professional fees. This revenue source ($449M in FY2014; *2*) primarily pays salaries of clinical faculty, but also helps to pay for hospital operations, management, and other clinical staff. The School of Medicine uses a small portion of professional-fee income, the so-called "Dean's tax" (~$25M in FY2014; *5*), for strategic projects and operational needs (see also chapter 8). Moreover, clinical departments and their divisions use small portions of their professional fee revenue to support their own faculty members' research and other activities (see chapter 9).

Other clinical revenue and educational activities. This grab-bag of revenues ($236M in FY2014; *1*) derives from and provides support for a variety of activities, including continuing education courses for health care providers, clinical support to some State prisons, small dental clinics in under-served neighborhoods, and—through the School of Medicine—a number of clinical services operated on a fee for service basis, including various clinics at San Francisco General Hospital, the UCSF Hemophilia Program, UCSF-Fresno programs, UCSF medical labs, and clinical operations of the Langley Porter Psychiatric Institute, plus affiliation agreements with other agencies, health care organizations and private health-related programs. Some revenues in this category even support a few genuinely "educational" activities (e.g., continuing education courses for clinicians and a small television channel). Little money in this category is available to support research, however.

Local government contracts. Local government agencies also sponsor agreements with UCSF ($156M in FY2014; *4*). While some of this money (~$20M) represents federal funds that flow through local non-federal government agencies to UCSF, most ($136M) of the total represents the contract between the City and County of San Francisco and UCSF to provide faculty and staff and assist in operation of San Francisco General Medical Center (*4*).

State educational appropriation. According to the state's constitution, the University of California (UC) is an independent entity with a governance structure largely independent from the state, with one crucial exception: UC has always received funding supplied by the state government and obtained by taxing its citizens. In 1979, the annual state education appropriation accounted for ~$67M, or 27% of UCSF's total revenues (then ~$250M; *6*); in FY2014 this appropriation ($198M; *1*) accounted for only 4.4% of UCSF's total revenues, and 10% of its Campus revenues. In 1979 dollars (*7*), the FY2014 sum would come to $47M—that is, 67% of its value 35 years earlier, when UCSF taught about the same number of students as it does now.

UCSF's decrease in state funding is paralleled on other UC campuses: in 17 of the 25 years between 1990 and FY2014, state support for the entire UC system decreased, limiting the overall increase in those 25 years to a meager 9% increase in nominal dollars, from ~$2.2B in 1990 to ~$2.4B in 2014 (*8*). In fact, the erosion is dramatically worse: if the 2014 state support appropriation instead had kept up with inflation (*7*) and with mandated increases in student enrollments, UC would have received ~$6.7B in state support in 2014—nearly three times the actual dollars appropriated in 2014 (*8*).

Auxiliary and other. Multiple enterprises—e.g., food service operations, student unions, parking operations and student and faculty housing systems—provide everyday services to UCSF's students, faculty, staff, and visitors. In FY2014, these enterprises earned revenues of $159M (*1*) or 8% of UCSF's Campus revenues. Auxiliary services sustain themselves financially (as they are required to do), owing to UCSF's large staff and faculty base. (Institutions with much larger student bases can sometimes use auxiliary services like these to contribute financially to the more general operation of the institution.) Within the "auxiliary" category at UCSF, patent income ($27M in FY2014; *1*) provides limited fungible revenue ($4.6M; *9*) for deans to distribute in UCSF's schools (predominantly the School of Medicine); the rest goes to faculty inventors and legal and administrative costs of patenting and licensing.

Student tuition and fees. The small number of students (3,094) who matriculate at UCSF provides revenues in the form of formal tuition and fees: $56M, or about 3% of Campus revenues in FY2014 (*1*). Tuition looms larger on UC campuses that teach more students, but at UCSF the entire amount is used to defray student-related costs UC forbids its schools to pay from state revenues, including non-educational "processing" of students (registration, admissions, financial aid, student counseling, and student health offices) and costs for student activities like student newspapers and legal aid. The $56M does not suffice to pay these costs, which must be subsidized from other revenues—leaving UCSF virtually zero tuition money to spend on actual education. Although UCSF does get a small amount of tuition money from professional school fees (called the PDST) in this total, the PDST was allowed by the State in the mid 1990's to replace State Educational funds that were being cut during that era of reductions.

Capital improvements. In addition to cutting education and operations, the state has decreased its contributions to capital improvements for UCSF even more dramatically (*10*). Until the early 1990s, the state was the predominant source of construction funds at UCSF, paying entirely for two research towers (1966) and the Ambulatory Care Center (1968), plus substantial proportions of costs for the new School of Dentistry (1980) and Long Hospital (1993), all on the Parnassus site. In the late 1970s UCSF began to receive small allocations of state capital funds: ~$10M annually, out of ~$250M for the UC system each year. Accelerated growth in numbers of undergraduates reduced UCSF's allocations still further in the 1990s, because its student numbers remained relatively low (*11*). From the late 1990s to now, the drought of state construction funds became more severe. UCSF's largest capital improvement, its Mission Bay research campus, cost ~$1.585B from 1997 to 2015 (*12*); of this cost, state capital funding contributed barely 4.8%, or $76M, including $21M toward the $215M construction of Genentech Hall, and $55M for the $95M QB3 building (*12*).

Steady reductions in capital funds and annual revenues supplied by the state required UCSF to become almost completely self-reliant in securing capital funds for constructing new teaching and research facilities (see chapter 4), and increasingly to depend on non-state sources to support education and research. UCSF still embraces its public service missions, but its identity as a "public institution" is much diluted.

Relative flexibility of different revenue streams. In summary, constraints on spending dollars accrued through different revenue streams vary considerably. UCSF has no flexibility in spending income from student tuition and fees, the auxiliary category, or most clinical revenues. Two revenue categories afford flexibility, but in small doses: (i) a relatively small "Dean's tax" (*5*) on professional fees for clinical care allows the Dean of the School of Medicine some opportunities for strategic spending and plugging holes in the budget (see above, and chapters 8 and 10, below); (ii) UCSF's schools and departments use 87% ($173M) of the state educational appropriation for salaries and benefits of faculty ($77M) and staff ($96M) who play roles in education, and $23M to pay for utilities and maintenance costs of teaching facilities (*13*). This much-reduced state appropriation pays only 15% of all UCSF faculty salaries (see chapter 6).

Several other revenue categories do furnish more flexibility: (i) partial reimbursements of certain "indirect" costs of research ($197M in FY2014; *4*), which the Chancellor controls (see chapters 3 and 5); (ii) ~$4.6M of patent

Table 2-1. UCSF endowments and gifts (FY2014)[*]

	Number	Principal ($M) (Totals)	Individual endowments	
			Median	Range
Total endowment				
Total[¶]	1,197	$1,987	$613K	$1K–$168M
New in FY2014	56	$38.5		
Non-endowment				
Gifts, FY2014[§]	31,129	$445		

*References *14*, *17*.
¶As of June 30, 2014.
§Reference *21*.

revenues provide a modest flexibility to the schools; (iii) endowments and gifts and other investment income provide further flexibility, subject to strong constraints, as discussed below.

Endowments and gifts

To thrive, and sometimes even to survive, academic institutions usually rely on the financial cushion of philanthropy. Gifts from individuals, foundations, and corporations can make crucial differences in UCSF's efforts to achieve world-class scientific discoveries, attract excellent faculty and students, and build first-class facilities for research and teaching. For many reasons, however, these gifts are no panacea.

Definitions. Table 2-1 summarizes gifts received by UCSF in FY2014 (*14*). Gifts—a term that includes endowments—may be given for specific or general purposes: e.g., to build a research laboratory, pursue a research program, support a faculty salary, stabilize institutional operating funds, etc. Gifts and endowments may have strings attached, but do not impose contractual requirements and are awarded irrevocably; unlike sponsored agreements, gifts do not require the institution to provide detailed technical reports or reports of expenditures (*15*). All endowments are gifts, but not all gifts are endowments, as we shall discuss in a moment.

At the end of FY2014, UCSF's 1,162 separate endowment funds added up to a total principal of ~$2B, and ranged in size over a wide range (Table 2-1; *15*, *16*). An endowment is a gift intended to provide long-term or even permanent value to the institution, and thus is usually a substantial cash gift whose principal is invested in long-term financial instruments that provide continuing income. Most private colleges and universities have "general endowments," which provide on-going income to help them pay general operating costs and salaries of teachers and support staff. For many years, UCSF neither had nor needed a general endowment, because it could rely on annual educational appropriations from the state. Instead, its departments, administrative units, or individual faculty solicited and received small endowments, given for more narrowly defined purposes—e.g., a lecture series or salaries (aka "chairs" and "professorships") for specific faculty. Now, like many other public institutions, UCSF badly needs more general endowment funds to make up for its reduced state educational appropriation.

Non-endowment gifts to UCSF. Gifts that are not endowments are usually given once and then spent for a specific item or activity. In FY2014, UCSF received a total of $445M in 31,129 non-endowment gifts (Table 2-1). The number of gifts is large, but most dollar amounts are relatively small: 89% of these amount to a total of ~$5M, or ~$185 per gift. A non-endowment gift can be used to construct a new building, renovate a laboratory, purchase equipment used in research or teaching, or support activities that advance an institutional mission or specific goal (e.g., funding an investigator's research aimed at treating infectious tropical diseases). Cash gifts donated for "general support of the institution" may be used for any legal purpose the institution chooses.

Large gifts ($20-50M or more) come with built-in constraints, which usually require a focus on a specific target, with little latitude for broader use. Thus the funding plan for a major capital endeavor, like the growing campus at Mission Bay, may include a large gift fund target, with major donors ultimately giving money to construct a specific building, but with little of the gift funds going into a general funding "pot" that pays for the entire program and its infrastructure. Moreover, large capital gifts are generally paid to UCSF over a period of 10 years or more, so the institution must borrow funds to "front" the money during construction and bear interest costs on the unpaid balance while the gift is paid incrementally. This "cost of doing business" dilutes the value of a large gift by 10-20%, depending on the size of the gift and the schedule of installments. Smaller cash gifts—e.g., for research lab renovations or costly research equipment—are usually paid up front, and the result is more

Table 2-2. UCSF's Endowments (Regents and UCSF Foundation), FY 2014*

	Regents	Foundation
All endowments		
Number[¶]	551	611
Principal (total, $M)	$1,082	$896
Net payout ($M)	$36.7	$31.6
Net payout rate (%)	3.4%	3.5%
Endowments with payout		
>$200K per year		
Number	37	16
Principal (total, $M)	$537	$317
% of total principal	49%	35%
Endowments with payout		
>$1M per year		
Number	4	1
Principal (total, $M)	$199	$173
% of total principal	18%	19%

*Data from references *14*, *16*, and *21*.

[¶]Reference 16. UCSF Development Office and Foundation finance director told one of the authors (on November 14, 2014) that there were 646 endowments in the Foundation at the end of FY 2014, but provided no subsequent substantiation from the Foundation financial reporting data. The finance director advised the authors on November 14, 2014, that the 35 missing endowments (= 646 - 611) had been "received" but not "set up". Since the FY 2014 financial data was never formally amended or changed, we chose to stick with the data we can validate.

immediate (within a few months to a year). In general, gifts to individual faculty contribute to UCSF's cash and balance sheet, but are for the most part unavailable for broader initiatives.

Rarely, a non-endowment gift directly funds research costs of an individual faculty member. UCSF looks closely into such "research support" gifts, to ensure that the money is a genuine gift, rather than an attempt to escape paying indirect costs (overhead) on what is really a sponsored agreement: a true gift is not subject to conditions imposed by the donor, nor does its receipt require written reports on its outcome (*15*). Gifts to individual faculty contribute to UCSF's cash and balance sheet, but are spent by those individuals and thus unavailable for broader initiatives.

Endowments and quasi-endowments. UCSF's endowments are held and managed by either of two parallel entities, the UC Regents or the UCSF Foundation (Table 2-2; *14*, *16*). The Regents controlled and conservatively invested all UC endowment funds until the mid-1980s, when UCSF and several other UC campuses petitioned them to allow individual campuses to raise and manage new gifts and endowments on their own. Agreeing, the Regents instituted controls to ensure fiduciary responsibility and management parallel to those of Regental endowments. The UCSF Foundation, like its counterparts at other campuses, is a corporation owned by the UC Regents and subject to Regental policies, but funded from and managed by UCSF. Compared to Regents' funds, the Foundation enjoys modestly greater flexibility and latitude for investment; critically, its returns from endowments can move into campus accounts within 30 days, vs. 3-6 months. As a bonus, the Foundation can set payouts from its investments at a slightly higher maximal level (5% vs. 4.75% for the Regents).

Actual "net" payout rates (Table 2-2) are lower than those maximal rates, for three reasons. (i) Rates are set to ensure that each year's payouts suffice to fund the targeted activity, while endowment principal keeps pace with inflation. To avoid sharp peaks and deep ravines in payouts in both flush and lean times (e.g., the major recession that began in 2008-9), fund managers apply "rate-smoothing," which averages capital gain or loss over periods of 3-5 years, so ravines become shallow valleys and sharp peaks become rolling hills. Inevitably, smoothing the recession's effects reduced payout rates, keeping them low in FY2014. (ii) Part of each payout (presently, just over half a 1% drop in the payout rate) helps to pay for administering the endowment. (iii) If the beneficiary unit (a department, school, or other endowed UCSF entity) does not need part of the fund's entire payout in a given year, it can request reinvestment of that part to increase the fund's principal.

The UCSF Foundation comes close to matching UCSF's share of Regental endowments in size and payouts (Table 2-2), and played essential roles in raising and managing cash gifts to pay for construction of the new campus at Mission Bay. UCSF's endowments, however, have not become maximally effective resources for funding flexible strategies or large new programs designed to accomplish academic missions of the Campus as a whole, because most of UCSF's separate endowment funds are extremely small, in both principal and payout (Table 2-2): in FY2014 less than half of all UCSF's individual endowment funds produced individual payouts greater than $200,000 per year, a sum that can barely sustain a substantial fraction of the salary and fringe benefits of a single senior faculty member; only five funds produced payouts greater than $1M per year (Table 2-2). Most small endowments (and their payouts) are under the control of academic departments or individual faculty members, rather than a larger entity able to use its payouts to benefit a wider spectrum of academic endeavor.

In FY2014, this decentralization left small portions of UCSF's total endowment principal under direct control of the Chancellor ($355M; 18% of the total) or the Dean of its largest School, Medicine ($315M; 16%). In fact, the bulk of the ~$12M and ~$10.5M annual payouts received from those funds by the Chancellor and the Dean, respectively, are devoted to ongoing operational needs (*17*). No problem when the state provided generous funding, decentralization now poses critical difficulties for a public university like UCSF, which lacks a general endowment usable for the entire institution's benefit.

For the Chancellor's office, this difficulty has been modestly mitigated by a "Chancellor's gift assessment." As the assessment was applied through June 2014, the Chancellor's office received 4% of the endowment principal at the time a gift was accepted, plus 1% of net annual payout, in addition to interest income earned on payout balances held by Schools, departments, or divisions—amounting, in FY2014, to a total of ~$17M (*18*). Beginning in July 2014, however, the Chancellor's "Infrastructure and Operations Fund" (IOF, for short) collects 4% at the time of receipt of each new gift or endowment principal and (by 2017, after a phasing-in period) 6% at the time expenditures from the campus gift or endowment account are posted. (One exception: these rules do not affect gifts restricted to paying tuition and living and other educational costs for students in degree programs.) The IOF's percentages are in keeping with similar practice at other research institutions (*18*), and their rationale is simple: over the next decade, without such an IOF, available sources will not suffice to meet projected demands for "funds that support the basic operations of the schools and administration, utilities, and infrastructure, and strategic campus wide initiatives" (*18*). While annual dollar totals of new gifts vary greatly from year to year, the new IOF arrangement will provide more than double the money received in FY2014—i.e., $35-40M per year (*18*), to be used for broad strategic purposes. (For further discussion, see chapter 4, below.)

One useful mechanism for strategic purposes is the "quasi-endowment" or a "Fund Functioning as an Endowment" (FFE). To create an FFE (which must be specifically approved by the Chancellor), an administrative entity at UCSF must identify a discretionary source of funding to be placed in an FFE and invested, via the UC Treasurer, in the UC General Endowment Pool, where it earns income and increases market capitalization (grows in size), just like an ordinary endowment. An FFE's key advantage is that its principal balance can be withdrawn and used as required. For example, the Chancellor's Instruction and Research Enrichment fund (CIRE fund), established in the mid-1990's and augmented from various sources, increased its principal balance to more than $25M by 2014, by capital growth and re-investment of annual payout. Almost all this FFE, plus an additional $4M of new gifts, was used to match a $30M gift from Michael Moritz and Harriet Heyman to establish a new Discovery Fellows Program (*19*), which helps to pay tuition and fees for graduate students. The Program's new FFE combines funds from the donors and the CIRE FFE.

The Chancellor can use a second (and even more limited) strategic mechanism, unrelated to endowments. UC's Office of the President (UCOP) authorizes the Chancellor to leverage UCSF's balance sheet for strategic purposes: the Chancellor can ask the UC Treasurer to invest up to 55% of cash available on UCSF's balance sheet (ceiling set by UCOP), to earn greater interest income in a Total Return Investment Pool (TRIP) than the same money can otherwise earn in a standard Short Term Investment Pool (STIP), which is nearly risk free. In this way, the Chancellor earned an "extra" ~$42M in FY2014— barely 2% of Campus revenue, but not an insignificant sum (*20*). Of this $42M, the Chancellor allocates ~$15M back to the School of Medicine and ~$3M to the Medical Center, representing their shares of the invested funds. The investment advantage is real: FY2014, 45% of UCSF's balance sheet, invested in TRIP, earned $42M; the remaining 55%, invested in STIP, earned only $14M; the Chancellor earned $31M more than the $11M that would have accrued if 100% had been invested in STIP.

Summary, so far

We have described in broad outline UCSF's revenue streams, endowments, and non-endowment gifts. These revenue sources add up to very large sums— $4.452B per year in revenues, endowment funds of nearly $2B, and non-endowment gifts of $445M per year. But most of these sources are already committed to pay for essential functions, leaving little fungible revenue for strategic academic purposes: that is, to educate students, pay a more substantial proportion of faculty salaries, or tackle new opportunities for research in basic biology or to combat disease.

A recent example is instructive. UCSF is correctly proud of its handling of one such recent opportunity, which began with the Moritz-Heyman gift ($30M) described above. UCSF combined this generous charitable gift with $29M from an FFE in the Chancellor's reserves, to produce a $59+M FFE—

now called the UCSF Discovery Fund— that will support graduate education. This apparently huge sum, $59M, comes to only 1.3% of UCSF's $4.452B budget, and only 3% of its Campus budget. Worse, the ~$2.24M yearly income from $59M (at a net payout of 4% per year) comes to only 6.8% of the ~$33M UCSF spends in tuition, fees, and stipends for basic science graduate students each year (for details, see chapter 8). Imagine what UCSF could do with three or ten times as much flexible money each year!

Our next chapter delineates the intricate and frustrating constraints, mixed with real opportunities, which accompany UCSF's strenuous efforts to recover dollars reimbursed for the indirect costs of research.

Chapter 3

Moiling for gold: The indirect cost mystery

Indirect cost recovery (ICR) seems easy to define: it is the dollars reimbursed to researchers' host institutions by funders of sponsored research projects, in order to pay the *indirect* costs institutions incur for research to take place. Although these indirect costs are incurred when research is actually performed, they are distinct from the *direct* costs (researcher salaries, supplies, etc.) of the research itself. Because indirect costs relate to facilities or administration, they are also called F&A costs. The F includes categories like utilities, laboratory maintenance and depreciation, and interest on loans to build research facilities; the A covers items like applying for research grants and supervising award expenditures, plus other research-related portions of university administration, ranging from the Chancellor to accounting and payroll, and more. This may sound straightforward, even humdrum, but dense clouds shroud ICR in mystery, controversy, and emotion at UCSF and most research institutions:

1. ICR, a glittering pot of gold, amounts to 9.5% of UCSF Campus revenues (*1*) and looms large in the academic imagination.
2. Access to this pot is especially valuable because its gold is relatively free of traditional or statutory obligations to narrowly defined university purposes. Access at UCSF is primarily the prerogative of the Chancellor, who uses it to guide ongoing efforts and support new projects and strategies, while other cash-hungry elements of the institution yearn to dip into the pot for their own purposes.
3. The glittering pot is shallow, because external funders fail to pay all indirect costs incurred. Nonetheless, universities eagerly seek more research funds from non-federal funders, although they pay smaller proportions of incurred indirect costs than does the federal government. Delving into its own coffers for dollars equivalent to 7.5% of Campus revenues, in FY2014 UCSF paid 46% of its incurred indirect costs.
4. Few administrators, and virtually no scientists, understand the maze of complex, arbitrary rules and calculations that make ICR so mysterious.

This chapter recounts the history of academic ICR, outlines federal rules for calculating indirect costs, shows how written and unwritten rules compel host institutions to share payment of actual indirect costs with federal and non-federal funding agencies, quantitates UCSF's indirect cost burden, and sketches dilemmas ICR poses for all research universities. Readers will begin to understand how ICR's complexity makes the cost recovery process resist change so strongly.

Before we proceed, a caveat: details of ICR at UCSF are not replicated at all academic research centers; each recovers a different proportion of the indirect costs it incurs, follows subtly different rules, and controls ICR revenues differently.

ICR: a pocket history

The practice of reimbursing universities for indirect costs was established during and after World War II, when the Office of Naval Research realized that contract research for special projects by university faculty could continue only if government were to pay indirect costs. In 1958 the principle of reimbursement, by then gradually adopted by other federal agencies, was formalized in Circular A-21, from the original Bureau of the Budget. The new ICR guidelines included criteria for justifying costs; rules and documentation requirements for distributing costs between research, instruction and other functions; and definitions of certain costs as unallowable on government research contracts. The Department of Health, Education, and Welfare, forerunner of today's Department of Health and Human Services (DHHS), initially set the rate for assessing indirect costs at a flat 8% of direct costs, but by 1966 the federal government replaced artificial indirect cost ceilings with a general policy that universities should be fully reimbursed for indirect costs incurred in conducting federal funded research projects. Simultaneous amendments to A-21, however, required universities to share paying the indirect costs of federal grants (e.g., by donating time of faculty or staff); A-21 also imposed new standards for compliance and documentation (2).

Since then Circular A-21 has been modified several dozen times, often to transform the initial cost sharing process into devices that trim federal reimbursement of indirect costs more effectively. Such devices restrict classes of direct costs for which indirect costs can be calculated; impose caps on certain indirect costs (e.g., researcher salaries); and demand that universities "negotiate" indirect cost rates with federal agencies. Together, they require most institutions to pay substantial shares of indirect costs from their own funds, and richly justify quotation marks for the verb, "negotiate."

From 1967 through 2011, UCSF's parent university, UC, comprehensively raided ICR generated on its campuses, keeping ~80% of their ICR revenue between 1967 and 1982. In FY1983, the office of UC's President (UCOP) finally began to relent, returning to UCSF 35% of the ICR it generated, and higher percentages to campuses with undergraduate students. UCSF's yearly "recovery" of its indirect costs from the parent university slowly improved thereafter, to more than 50% in 2000; by FY2012, UCOP was returning 100% of ICR generated at UCSF, as well as its other campuses (Fig. 3-1, *3*) Over the years, UCOP consumed several hundred million dollars of research indirect costs earned at UCSF. The ICR battle between UC and its research campuses exemplifies academia's ceaseless lust for control of indirect cost reimbursement.

Calculating indirect costs—aka: quantifying muddles

After a restaurant meal, customers pay two bills: the restaurant's price for each dish consumed, plus a gratuity for the waiter. The first cost requires a "rational" market decision, weighing anticipation of the meal's quality against menu prices. The gratuity decision is arbitrary and uncertain, however, with respect

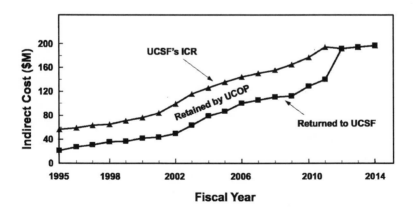

Fig. 3-1. Indirect costs "earned" by UCSF or returned to UCSF (red) after UCOP removed a share for its own purposes. Dollars between the two lines were "retained" by UCOP. Data from *4*.

both to the amount to be paid and the customer's ignorance of where the dollars may go (to the waiter, alone? shared with other waiters? or with dishwashers and cooks, as well?). The reality: restaurants don't pay waiters enough to keep them working, so diners are asked to pay waiters a percentage of the bill. Restaurants are not universities, and diners pay for food rather than research, but the menu-specified price closely resembles a "direct cost," in that buyers know how much to pay and what they will get in return. Gratuities share two key characteristics with indirect costs for research: (i) the actual amounts to be paid are fraught with mystery and muddlement, for both payer and payee, but (ii) if the gratuity or indirect cost is not paid, the direct-cost transaction will not work.

In universities the imprecision of indirect costs reflects the fact that virtually every employee (administrator, faculty member, janitor, etc.) and every building's square feet, electric wires, or heating ducts contribute to multiple functions—i.e., teaching, research, and, at UCSF, patient care. This mixing makes it impossible to trace or count dollars paid for each contribution, so indirect costs are usually allocated as a percentage of the direct cost, like gratuities. The rules governing that percentage are vastly complex, inevitably arbitrary, and often unfair, albeit to unknown degrees.

Assessing indirect costs is a prime example of the critical (but usually ignored) Muddlement-Uncertainty Principle, or M-UP (4). In its simplest form, the M-UP states that irretrievably muddled mixing of categories prevents analysts from quantifying financial facts with the degree of accuracy desired—or even needed—to drive key decisions. The M-UP affects analysis of every financial transaction of every academic research center and most large businesses and institutions. In its more general form, the M7-UP, the keyword muddlement may be replaced by Multiplicity, Mystery, and Mistakes, and (at least with respect to the US federal budget) by Magic, Mendacity, and even Malevolence. For academic ICR, muddlement alone typically suffices.

Although UCSF receives sponsored dollars—for both direct and indirect costs—from several kinds of sources, our account of indirect cost calculations starts by focusing on federally funded research, which accounts for most (73%) of UCSF's *recovered* indirect costs (Table 3-1; 5). We must distinguish between ICR rates and the actual *amount* of indirect cost incurred, including the part that is reimbursed and the part that is not. Careful analysis of the actual amount of incurred indirect costs serves as the starting point for the negotiations between the institution and federal auditors that determine ICR rates as a percentage of indirect costs, relative to direct costs:

Table 3-1. Indirect costs recovered in FY2014*

Category	Direct costs ($M)	Indirect costs ($M)	% of Non-fed	% of all recovered
Federal	$507	$144	—	73%
Non-federal				
State	57	9	17	4
Local	19	2	4	1
Priv. clinical trials	22	6	11	3
Priv. grants, contracts	190	36	67	19
Non-federal total	$288	$53	100%	27%
Total (Fed + Non-fed)	$795	$197	—	100%

*Data from *5*, but contracts with affiliated hospitals for medical services have been excluded; although these contracts reflect direct costs paid to UCSF in sponsored contracts, they neither represent costs of research nor were ever proposed (by UCSF or anyone else) as subject to "recovery" of indirect costs.

ICR rate (%) = [total indirect costs ÷ direct costs] x 100

To establish the amount of indirect costs (and subsequently an ICR rate), an academic institution must first show the federal government, in detail, how it defines and identifies the indirect costs it actually incurs, by a process that costs so much that universities can afford to tackle it only every four years or so. Based on existing federal allocation formulas, however, the complex definition-and-identification exercise (Box 3-1) probably does approximate (a version of) the "truth," despite the muddled categories it dissects.

Throughout the exercise, UCSF's analysts are keen to ensure that the documented indirect cost pools they assess do not generate complications like the brouhaha triggered by Stanford University's difficulty with federal auditors 25 years ago (*8*). Stanford did not write a check from federal funds to pay for maintaining either a yacht or Leland Stanford's tomb, but *did* fail to remove these costs from the indirect cost "pools" it used to calculate and then negotiate the ICR rate—thereby violating a federal law that prohibits false claims for

Box 3-1. Calculating incurred indirect costs of research at UCSF

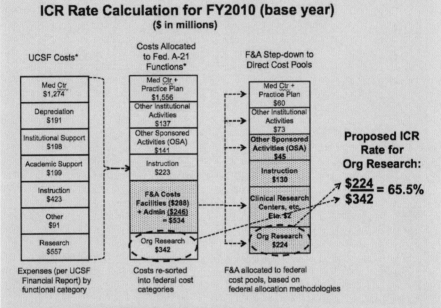

Fig. 3-2. The ICR rate calculation, controlled by federal rules and allocation formulas involves three stages, each depicted in the vertical columns and described in the Box.

Figure 3-2 shows the process by which UCSF calculated UCSF's indirect research costs for FY2010, which was the base year for its most recent negotiation with federal auditors. The calculation's complexity reflects a brave attempt to combat the M-UP (Muddlement Uncertainty Principle; main text), even when details are stripped to a bare minimum. Proceeding from left to right, the Figure's vertical columns depict three sequential stages of the calculation, each dictated by federal guidelines and (for FY2010), extensively reviewed by federal auditors. To make the process work, UCSF's general ledger system had to be able to account for and classify all the university's costs into categories that will ultimately be assigned to direct and indirect cost pools (6) specified and allocated by detailed federal guidelines. Those categories differ sharply from the usual parsing of expenses into salary plus benefits, supplies, travel, etc.

The first stage of the process (left column) divides all UCSF's expenditures in FY2010 into straightforward categories defined by the common accounting lexicon for all universities. These categories include both direct and indirect operating costs, but exclude those not allowed by federal rules, so reducing the year's total expenditures ($3,179M) to $2,933M by removing $246M in unallowable costs—that is, expenditures that failed to qualify as Modified Direct Costs (MTDC; see main text).

The next step re-sorts all expenditures from UCSF's ledger into five federally-defined direct cost categories (white boxes in the figure's middle column), plus the facilities and administrative (F&A) indirect cost category (highlighted box, middle column). This re-sorting followed detailed formulas specified by the federal government. Total dollars in the middle and left columns are identical, so no middle-column category is defined with respect to sources that supplied its dollars. Expenditures in the Instruction category, for example, included not only instruction paid for by external grants or contracts, but also instruction funded by UCSF, by tuition and fees, or by UC (as if the latter were a kind of "external sponsor" of education for medical and other professional students). Similarly, Organized Research (OR) costs include dollars supplied by federal or non-federal sources, or by UCSF itself (which pays, for instance, portions of some researchers' salaries). F&A costs in this column include facilities and administration for all UCSF missions (not just research); part, but by no means all, of these F&A costs were paid from indirect costs reimbursed by external sponsors.

Next comes the "F&A step-down" process, aimed at determining which proportions of the total F&A indirect cost pool (in the central column) are associated with each of the six "direct cost" pools listed in the right-hand column. This step-down analysis and calculations are also based on a series of complex federally-specified allocation formulas and rules. In general, the facilities portion of F&A related to a particular direct cost pool depends on the space occupied by that direct-cost pool's activities (e.g., by research in a particular subunit, department, or division of UCSF, in proportion to the subunit's total space); similarly, that F&A pool's administrative component usually depends on the "direct-cost" expenditures of the UCSF subunit, as a proportion of its total expenditures. In every case, federal auditors carefully reviewed both data and calculations. In no case is all the F&A related to a particular direct cost pool subject to reimbursement by any external funding agency: the two white boxes in the right-hand column, clearly UCSF's responsibility, involve no F&A recovery from external sources; some portion of F&A in each of the column's four highlighted boxes, however, may be recovered from external sources.

The last step of the process is to calculate the indirect cost rate UCSF will propose for each direct cost function in order to recover the corresponding indirect costs from external funders; rates are calculated in the four highlighted categories: Organized Research (OR), instruction, and Other Sponsored Activities (OSA). The example in this figure calculates the F&A indirect cost rate, as a percentage, by dividing the proposed F&A amount for OR by the direct cost (actually, the MTDC) of OR, and multiplying the result by 100. UCSF began its 2012 negotiations with DHHS auditors by justifying and proposing this percentage as the calculated indirect cost rate for OR. As described in the text, however, federal negotiators offered a much lower rate for OR. Regardless of negotiation, proposed rates in other highlighted categories would not have recouped many dollars in the way of indirect cost recovery, as compared to OR, because these categories were not associated with large amounts of direct costs (7).

reimbursement. (For a partial list of other "unallowable" indirect costs, see 9.) In 1991, the resulting publicity helped to support tighter federal restrictions and documentation requirements, plus a 26% cap on the administrative portion of all university indirect cost rates (see below, and 10).

Once indirect cost pools are purged of unallowable costs and calculated, the university is ready to defend the ICR rate it proposes for negotiation. But the federal government requires that the direct costs used for that calculation not include all the dollars (Total Direct Costs, or TDC) in the awarded grant or contract. Instead, TDC must be reduced to MTDC (Modified TDC, or MTDC), which specifically excludes certain direct expenses—e.g., for equipment, patient care, rental of off-campus space, graduate training stipends and tuition, and sub-contract costs greater than $25,000. Substituting MTDC for TDC, the equation becomes:

ICR rate (%) = [total indirect costs ÷ MTDC] x 100

Universities and federal agencies hotly debated the substitution of MTDC for TDC before it was instituted in 1979, for good reason. Some MTDC-driven exclusions are logical and reasonable, and others not, but their overall effect, at any fixed ICR rate, will always limit the federal dollars reimbursed for indirect costs by institutions; that is, if ICR rates already being applied remain constant, substituting the lower MTDC figure as the divisor in the equation above must inevitably reduce the actual dollar amount of ICR by universities. Over the 35 subsequent years, however, negotiated ICR rates and ICR amounts have changed substantially. At UCSF, for example, the ICR rate on federal grants for "Organized Research" (OR) more than doubled (from 27.5% in 1982 to 57% in 2014; *11*); the dollar *amount* of recovered indirect costs on all of UCSF's federal grants increased about seven-fold during almost exactly the same period (FY1985-FY2014; see 3, *12*). Thus the old MTDC argument is no longer relevant. Instead, as we shall see, the pivotal decision about the amount of indirect costs to be reimbursed/recovered is made when federal auditors and the institution negotiate a new set of indirect cost recovery *rates*, about every four years. Each institution proposes those new ICR rates based on documented *amounts* of both MTDC and F&A costs incurred by the institution in the year prior to expiration of previously negotiated rates (Box 3-1). The real problems with recovering indirect costs arise at later steps of the process, including the negotiation itself.

Before negotiation begins, institutional proposals for ICR rates are reviewed by auditors appointed by the federal executive branch—DHHS for UCSF—that funds most of the its grants and contracts. For 3-6 months DHHS auditors review hundreds of pages documenting UCSF's direct and indirect operating costs and proposal for new ICR rates. Then they visit UCSF for several more months, to inspect facilities, interview staff and researchers, and check UCSF's proposal against financial and other records. Finally, the panel "negotiates" with the Chancellor's Department of Budget and Finance to determine the actual ICR rate. (Later, we sketch the course of a recent negotiation.)

The last step in the process, actual recovery of incurred indirect costs, takes place only after UCSF's researchers pay *direct* research costs by spending awarded grant or contract dollars: applying appropriate negotiated ICR rates to these payouts, UCSF requests reimbursement from the federal funding agency several times a week; the agency usually pays each incremental indirect cost bill within 24 hours. (Thus ICR on federal grants is paid only when and if dollars are actually spent from those grants.)

Unrecovered ICR on federal grants in FY2014

Some researchers assume that ICR payments from funders of direct costs cover *all* indirect costs incurred by the university in support of research. Not so. Instead, in FY2014 UCSF recovered $144M in indirect costs on all its federally sponsored research projects; but this represented only 64% of the $226M in federal indirect costs incurred in that year, so that UCSF was obliged to pay the remaining 36% ($82M) from its own coffers (Table 3-2; *13*).

Table 3-2. Federal indirect costs: Incurred, recovered, and unrecovered in FY2014

	$M	% of all unrec.	% of all incurred
Recovered*	$144	—	64%
Unrecovered¶			
Caps	37.5	46	16
Cost sharing	3	4	2
Negotiation	26	32	11
Grant type	15.5	18	7
Total	$82	100%	36%
Incurred§ (= recovered + all losses)	$226	—	100%

*Data from 13.

§Incurred indirect costs were calculated exactly as described in Box 3-1, except that the incurred F&A costs in each grant or contract subcategory were calculated by multiplying the actual FY2014 MTDC amounts in the subcategory by the percentage for total F&A UCSF proposed (at the start of its negotiations with federal auditors in 2012) for that category for FY2014. Thus the "incurred" dollars are based on (i) actual MTDC amounts in FY2014 (5) and (ii) UCSF's specification of F&A in FY2014. (Federal auditors did negotiate for lower percentages, but audited and did not dispute UCSF's numbers.) The total amount of calculated/incurred F&A ("computed recovery") for federal grants in FY2014 was $226M; in that year UCSF actually recovered $144M on federally-funded projects, so that the (unrecovered) deficit on federal ICR comes to $82M, as shown in the Table.

¶Dollar values of unrecovered indirect costs were derived as follows:

Caps of two kinds: (i) Administrative. The federal government (OMB) implemented a cap on the administrative component of all university ICR rates of 26%. Any amount above the 26% cap is calculated at the start of each rate negotiation process and can't be recovered from the federal government. UCSF calculated its administrative component at 6% over the 26% cap. The cost of a rate decrease of 1% in 2014 was just over $3.5M (6% X $3.5M = $21M). (ii) On salary level (>$185,000) of faculty and staff. Any amount above this threshold cannot be charged to federal contracts and grants. The UCSF Controller's office computes this amount at the end of each fiscal year based on actual salary costs ($16.5M for 2014).

Cost sharing. This amount, $3M for 2014, computed by the UCSF Controller's Office at fiscal year's end, is based on actual cost sharing identified in the general ledger.

Negotiation. This amount is the 11.5% difference between UCSF's Facilities rate calculation and the rate agreed to by federal negotiators, which amounted to $26M total because each rate point difference was worth just over $3.5M (see just above).

Grant type. This adds up to $15.5M of unrecovered indirect costs, all related to multiple, hard-to-list/describe-in-detail variations in indirect costs federal rules allow universities to charge in relation to different kinds of grants—to, in other words, the M-UP's ineluctable complexity. Examples: (i) In 2014, UCSF's portfolio of federal agreements still included very many contracts and grants for projects whose indirect costs were negotiated in earlier years when the OR rate was lower than the 57% OR rate negotiated in 2012, for grants to be awarded in the future. (ii) The off-campus OR rate is set at 26%; (iii) NIH mandates reimbursement of universities' indirect costs at a fixed 8% rate on instruction/training grants (well below most universities' negotiated instruction rates). We elected not to lure readers into the M-UP jungle by trying to define and calculate incurred indirect costs for more than a dozen specialized grant categories. Instead, readers may rest assured that these numbers of unrecovered dollars for different grant types ($15.5M total), plus the dollars unrecovered because of caps, cost sharing, and negotiation, add up to the $82M difference for federal grants between the calculated/incurred $226M described above (see note§) and the recovered $144M actually recovered.

For federal contracts and grants, the difference between incurred and recovered indirect costs reflects four classes of lost ICR revenue, each created by explicit regulations and/or traditional and effectively non-negotiable practice.

Lost ICR (i): different ICR rates for different types of research grant. Academic researchers tend to cite on-campus Organized Research (OR) rates—which UCSF negotiated earlier to be 57% for FY2014—as if the OR rate applied to all federal grants, but this is not the case. For instance, in its contract with DHHS UCSF negotiated an ICR rate of 44% for instruction grants, but NIH refuses to honor that rate and advised the institution that to be awarded a training grant it must accept an 8% rate. NIH also sets special rates for different components of federal grants like those that support UCSF's Clinical and Translational Science Institute (CTSI); finally, UCSF negotiates an Other Sponsored Activity (OSA) rate (34%) for federal grants and contracts that do not fit into OR or instructional categories. (Some NIH institutes have begun to set their own ICR rates for specific types of research, but not yet so consistently that UCSF finds it worthwhile to track ICR lost in this way.) Overall, these special rates, among which the very low rate on training grants did the most damage, cost UCSF $15.5M in FY2014 (Table 3-2). While ICR based on the negotiated OR rate (57%) accounts for the bulk of UCSF's federally reimbursed revenues, blending OR recovery from federally funded grants with the lower recovery for training and a few other types of grants dilutes UCSF's overall effective federal recovery rate to ~41% (5); the loss would be higher if graduate training represented larger proportions of UCSF's NIH grants.

Lost ICR (ii): caps on certain classes of expenditures. The federal government also places ceilings or caps on specific kinds of research expenses for which ICR can be charged. UCSF's Finance office calculates that in FY2014 the combination of two such caps caused the institution to lose $37.5M in unrecovered ICR (Table 3-2):

a. A 26% cap on administrative costs (instituted in 1991, after the famous indirect cost audit debacle at Stanford; *8*) caused UCSF in FY2014 to lose ~$21M; Table 3-2). That loss represents a decrease of 6 percentage points from the administrative ICR rate (32% of MTDC) UCSF calculated and proposed in 2012 to the federal auditors, who did not question UCSF's figures. Touted as a way to promote more efficient research administration, this cap ignores the gradual increase in universities' administrative burdens that results from having to comply with the ever-growing flood of regulations crafted by federal funders (*14*). Such compliance costs, reflected in increasing administrative rate calculations, have dramatically increased, but have not yet been comprehensively assessed by at a national level (e.g., by the Council on Governmental Relations or the Association of American Universities).

b. A cap on maximum individual salaries that may be paid as direct costs by NIH-funded projects. In FY2014, universities were required to use other sources of income to pay the portion of faculty salaries above that cap (set at $181,500 per year, a pay grade for certain federal employees). Annual extra cost to UCSF: ~$16.5M (Table 3-2).

c. The NIH-mandated 8% ICR rate on training grants, described above under i, represents another kind of cap specified by federal agencies. (This kind of cap did not contribute to the $37.5M in ICR lost under headings a and b, above.)

Lost ICR (iii): cost sharing by faculty. UCSF advises its investigators not to participate in voluntary (but unpaid) sharing of direct costs, but some faculty members still do so. Thus Professor X, a leader in her field, may promise to donate 5% of her time to Assistant Professor Y's project, with no salary requested; such voluntary participation may make the proposal look stronger to reviewers who decide whether to fund it. If X keeps her promise, the university must pay 5% of X's salary from other sources. UCSF records the overall cost of this voluntary sharing as $3M in FY2014 (Table 3-2).

Lost ICR (iv): "negotiation." Negotiation with DHHS auditors substantially decreases UCSF's recovery of federal ICR (Table 3-2). Various institutions get quite different negotiated ICR rates, sometimes because they negotiate with different government agencies or come to the table as a private research institute (with no mission other than research) rather than as an academic institution. Different histories can account for some discrepancies: for instance, generous state support for public universities through the 1980s kept ICR rates lower than for private institutions. Subsequent loss of much of that state support gradually helped UCSF to negotiate higher ICR rates (compare the 57% negotiated OR rate in FY2014 to the 42% OR rate in FY1994 (11); even so, UCSF's OR ICR rates do not yet match those of institutions whose ICR rates were much higher early on. In other cases, reasons for different negotiated rates remain unexplained (15).

UCSF last negotiated with federal auditors in 2012, when its negotiated OR rate was 54.5% (26% administrative; 28.5% facilities), based on rates negotiated previously. To the auditors UCSF proposed new OR rates, based on federally audited UCSF expenditures in the index year of FY2010 (see Box 3-1). The proposed OR rate was 71.3% for FY2013, dropping to 70% over the ensuing four years. For each year, the proposal asked for a 32% rate to pay its administrative component. At the very outset the 26% federal cap for administration automatically reduced the ICR rate for OR by 6%.

The rest of the negotiation revolved around the difference between the 2011 facilities rate (28.5%) and UCSF's proposed 40% facilities rate, or 11.5% higher. The proposed increase was based on a combination of new costs for two recently occupied new research buildings and two additional buildings to be opened during the four years to be covered by the proposed new rate; the increased costs included interest on new bonds, building depreciation, and utilities, operations, and maintenance. Without arguing against the basis for the proposed increase, DHHS auditors simply offered a gradual 4% increase in the facilities rate—take it or leave it. Because the alternative would have been to give up NIH-funded research, UCSF accepted the offer (16). "Negotiation" thus meant UCSF itself, not NIH, had to pay the unrecovered 7.5% from the facilities component of its ICR rate, a loss of ~$26M per year (Table 3-2). In FY2015, the negotiated OR rate is 58%; UCSF is preparing for another rate negotiation in 2016, which will presumably cover fiscal years 2017-20.

ICR on non-federal research grants and contracts

In actual dollars, recovery of indirect costs for federally sponsored research was almost three-fold higher in FY2014 than that for non-federally sponsored research—$144M vs. $53M, respectively (Table 3-1; Fig. 3-3). As we saw in chapter 1 (see Fig. 1-5), research funds from private funding sources have increased mightily, especially since the beginning of the 21st century. This increase reflects enthusiastic and effective efforts of clinician-researchers to garner more privately funded support (see chapter 9). Consequently, recovered indirect cost dollars for privately funded research have also risen during the same period (Fig. 3-3).

Nonetheless, increased private research funds do pose a problem. If we compare recovery in proportion to total direct costs, funders of federal research also reimburse at a higher rate than do non-federal funders: for the two, ratios of the recovered indirect costs to the total direct costs in FY 2014 were 0.28 and 0.18, respectively. The different reimbursement rates probably reflect two causes. First, the reimbursement policies of many important private sponsors of academic research (e.g., American Cancer Society or the American Heart Association) explicitly limit the percentage of indirect cost they will pay, to assure donors that their donations will directly fund research. Some corporate sponsors do pay at rates comparable to federal rates, although privately sponsored clinical trials reimburse at a special rate of 33%, set by the UCSF Chancellor's Office (levied on TDC, rather than MTDC; *17*). The second cause is an essential corollary to the first: like most large biomedical research centers, UCSF usually waives its stated policy that non-federal funders pay indirect costs at the federal rate. Indeed, federal rules require grantee institutions to charge indirect costs to non-federal funders at federal rates, but also allow them to waive such charges if they set up a formal waiver process. UCSF formally waives a large proportion of the non-federal indirect costs it would otherwise charge. The waivers reflect market decisions parallel to the institution's acceptance of the "negotiated" loss of indirect costs on federally sponsored grants (see above). In both cases, UCSF recognizes its weak bargaining position: to obtain direct costs necessary for research, it must absorb unavoidable deficits in unrecovered indirect costs.

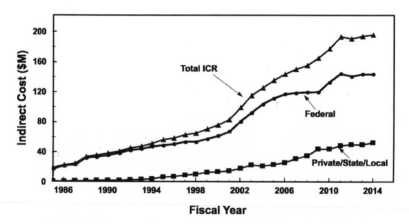

Fig. 3-3. Indirect costs recovered by UCSF over thirty years (1985-2014): total ICR; federal ICR; non-federal, or Private, State, and Local ICR. Data from *12*).

Because the proportion of UCSF's non-federal research dollars to its total research dollars increases every year, it may be useful to quantitate the unrecovered indirect costs the university itself pays to receive non-federal research support. To determine that number, in turn, requires an estimate of the total indirect costs actually *incurred* when UCSF accepts grants and contracts from non-federal sponsors. That estimate has remained distressingly fuzzy, because UCSF does not request or receive most of its indirect costs from non-federal funders in relation to federally-specified cost-allocation categories, nor does it track indirect costs specifically related to non-federally-funded research grants.

To manage this fuzziness, we take advantage of the fact that federal rules require that its allocation categories be applied to UCSF expenditures for all research, not only to that funded by federal sources (Box 3-1). Because research funded by both federal and non-federal sponsors takes place in the

Table 3-3. Non-federal indirect costs: Incurred, recovered, and unrecovered in FY2014

	$M	% of all unrec.	% of all incurred
Recovered*	$53	——	39%
Unrecovered[§]			
State C&G	18	22	13
Local C&G	7	9	5
Private clinical trials	4	5	4
Private C&G	53	64	39
Total	$82	100%	61
Incurred[¶]	$135	—	100%

*Data from 5.

¶Total incurred indirect costs were calculated according to the same MTDC-based procedure (see legend to Table 3-2) used for calculating federally funded contracts and grants (C&G). They were then distributed into four categories based on the relative direct costs (MTDC) received from four classes of non-federal funding agency (state, local, private) and the kind of research (private clinical trials, private C&G); these distributed incurred costs are not shown in this table.

§Unrecovered indirect costs were calculated by subtracting the actual indirect costs reimbursed from each funder category from the calculated incurred indirect costs (not shown, but see footnote above) in that category.

same facilities, is performed by the same researchers, and is administered by the same staff, it appears likely that indirect costs incurred for non-federal research closely resemble those for federal research. We used federal allocation categories to calculate the incurred indirect costs in FY2014 for federally-sponsored research (Table 3-2), so applying similar rules to non-federally sponsored research should provide an equally valid result. The key assumption is this: the non-federal MTDC dollar generates quantitatively the same *incurred* indirect cost at UCSF as does a federal MTDC dollar. Subsequent subtraction of ledger-recorded *recovered* indirect costs from the calculated incurred costs can then tell us the amounts of *unrecovered* indirect costs in each subcategory of non-federal research.

Table 3-3 shows the results based on these assumptions. For non-federal research, in FY2014 UCSF recovered $53M of the $129M it incurred, and failed to recover $76M. Most of these unrecovered costs —$49M, or 64%— could be attributed to privately sponsored research contracts and grants, and relatively little to unrecovered funds in other subcategories.

Earlier we suggested that the M-UP makes indirect cost calculations— even those that obey the federal government's precisely prescribed rules— quantitatively imprecise approximations of reality. Extrapolating these rules to non-federally sponsored research must add yet more uncertainty, because we do not know for sure whether indirect costs of federally- vs. non-federally-funded research are muddled in exactly the same way. Despite the caveats, dollar amounts in the section below are as nearly correct as the M-UP allows.

Overall IC recovered vs. IC incurred

Rough estimates of UCSF's incurred indirect costs of research in FY2014 (Fig. 3-4) yield three useful pieces of information about how UCSF pays for its research:

1. *UCSF's overall research effort costs nearly half the total revenues of its Campus* (Fig. 3-4a). The sum of total direct costs of sponsored research ($795M; Table 3-1) and the total calculated/estimated indirect costs incurred ($361M; Tables 3-2 and 3-3) comes to $1,156M, or 47% of UCSF's Campus revenues ($2,480M; *1*).

2. *From its own resources, UCSF pays nearly half the indirect costs its research incurs* (Fig. 3-4b). The incurred indirect costs of all sponsored research ($361M) vastly exceeded the $197M reimbursed by all funders, producing an indirect cost deficit of $164M, or 45% of all indirect

costs and a deficit burden that is 7.5% of UCSF's total annual Campus revenue.

3. *For UCSF, federally funded research is a substantially better financial bargain than non-federally funded research.* Despite 12 years of flat-lined NIH budgets, UCSF received 64% of its total sponsored research direct costs ($507M) from federal sources—almost double the 36% ($288M) received from non-federal sources (Fig. 3-4a). But funders of the two classes of research failed to reimburse exactly the same amounts ($82M each; a fortuitous coincidence) of Indirect costs (Fig. 3-4b). Consequently, UCSF was obliged to pay 61% of incurred indirect costs of non-federal research, but only 36% of those incurred in supporting federal research.

The third piece of information indicates that non-federally funded research can create a distressing dilemma for UCSF, and presumably for other large academic biomedical research centers. As the NIH budget shrank (in inflation-corrected dollars; *18*) by 21% from FY2003 to FY2014 (*19*), UCSF and its sister institutions continued to scramble furiously for research funding from philanthropic and other non-federal sources. (Also corrected for inflation, non-federally-funded research at UCSF increased 5.5-fold, vs. 2.4-fold for federally-funded research over the much longer period, 1984 to 2013; see Chapter 1, Fig. 1-5b.) But in FY2014, the lower recovery of indirect costs on non-federally funded research requires UCSF to pay 29 cents on average for each non-federal direct cost dollar—that is, 13 cents more than it pays per federal direct cost dollar (*20*). If the swerve toward more non-federal support for research continues, universities like UCSF will find themselves unable to bear the growing financial burden.

Why do UCSF and its sister schools tolerate these fiscally painful burdens, whether they involve federal or non-federal funders? Are these schools helplessly trapped between faculty lusting for money to support their research and penny-pinching federal and non-federal sponsors powerful enough to call the shots? The trap metaphor captures only part of the problem, which is really historical: during the latter half of the 20th century many leading US universities, including the University of California, began to take on a new mission, in addition to educating the young—that is, production of new knowledge (*21*). Now, after more than six decades, employees of those universities—from lowly wage-workers to top leaders—take genuine pride in their institutions' research accomplishments, which attract excellent students, superb faculty, and millions of dollars from alumni, philanthropists, foundations, corporations, and government. Because their jobs and future prospects depend directly on

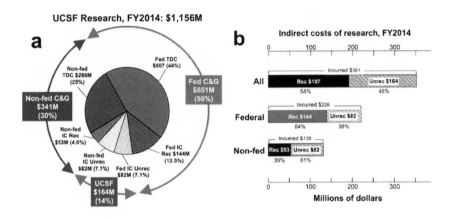

Fig. 3-4 a & b. Dollars spent on research at UCSF (panel a) and indirect costs of research (panel b) in FY2014. Sections of the pie in panel a are associated with federal or non-federal grants and contracts. Outer arcs and arrows indicate proportions of total research dollars according to pay source: federal, non-federal, or UCSF itself. Indirect costs in panel b are separated into two categories: recovered; unrecovered; the horizontal bars depict indirect costs of (from bottom to top) non-federally-funded research, federally funded research, and all research in that year. Abbreviations: Fed, federal; non-fed, non-federal; C&G, contracts and grants; TDC, total direct costs; IC, indirect costs; Rec, recovered; Unrec, unrecovered. All data derived from Tables 3-1-3.

these accomplishments, institutional sharing of research's indirect costs with government and non-federal sponsors remains a necessary and tolerated—albeit poorly understood—bargain. While febrile eagerness to keep that bargain induces institutions to invest ever-increasing dollars into research, the substantial benefits and potential dangers of sharing the indirect costs of research will continue to raise additional concerns. These dangers are surely accentuated by progressively decreasing willingness of the public and state and federal government funders to maintain—let alone increase—past levels of funding, both direct and indirect.

Indirect costs pose other difficult questions

For what purposes may universities legitimately spend ICR revenue? Researchers often raise this question, mostly to urge that every dime of that revenue directly supports research, and more particularly, research in their own laboratories. Nonetheless, no university- or sponsor-generated regulations contradict the principle that the institution—at UCSF, the Chancellor's Office—can use ICR dollars for any purpose in keeping with university missions, because those dollars are reimbursed to the university for real costs already incurred. Employers reimburse employees for costs incurred in pursuing business purposes: reimbursement to an employee who uses her car to travel to a business meeting requires documentation of trip and meeting, but she is not required to spend the reimbursement check on her car, or for any other specific purpose. Thus universities may use ICR dollars to support research, but are not required to do so. UCSF Chancellors generally follow an unwritten policy of using the ICR dollars to support research and education. Chapter 5 will return to these issues.

Institutions jump through fiery hoops to garner whatever indirect cost reimbursements funders deign to provide, because they want to pursue research and need every dollar they can get to survive and prosper. These straightforward facts raise yet more questions. We pose them here, so readers can ponder the underlying issues before they re-appear in later chapters:

1. Given UCSF's pressing need for indirect cost reimbursements, do federal rules for calculating those reimbursements skew institutional incentives in directions that make it harder to maintain the high qualify of biomedical research? Bruce Alberts pointed out (22) that universities are motivated against paying substantial proportions of faculty researchers' salaries, because faculty salaries paid from grants constitute much of the MTDC to which ICR rates are pegged. Indeed, if UCSF itself had paid all faculty researcher salaries charged to research grants in FY2014, it would not only have had to pony up an extra $114M in direct salary and $34M in benefits, but would also have lost an additional ~$60M in ICR—a total of $208M. [These sums derive from: (i) dollars of direct sponsored faculty salaries (see chapter 6); (ii) benefits calculated as 29.7% of that sponsored salary; (iii) 41% ICR on direct costs of federal grants.] Faced with the federal ICR rules on researcher salaries, a university leader who proposes that his institution pay a higher proportion of researchers' salaries might well be judged insane.
2. Do universities continue to build or renovate laboratories—as Alberts also suggested (22)—because the government allows ICR to pay the interest on money borrowed to do so? For UCSF, this incentive is real, but relatively weak (see Chapter 4).

Finally, let us pose a question that should occur to almost any observer. How does a university find dollars to pay for all its unrecovered indirect costs? For

UCSF, the shortfall of indirect cost reimbursement was ~\$164M in FY2014 (Fig. 3-4a), including both federally- and privately-sponsored research grants. Where did UCSF find the dollars to pay this money, especially in view of progressively declining support from UC and the state of California? The short answer: no one, including the authors of this book, can provide a straightforward quantitative answer.

The long answer: the M-UP strikes again! In essence, the dollars for every activity that involves research in any large academic institution are muddled irretrievably with everything else the university does. So, as we described above, calculating total incurred indirect costs produces an estimate, for which the arithmetic is easy to record and check (e.g., by federal auditors), although its true accuracy can never be known. From the very beginning of "indirect costs," no "real" unrecovered indirect cost of research has ever been tracked and used as a basis of negotiation with any research funding source. When indirect costs were first paid, sophisticated data systems able to track such information didn't exist, and no one imagined requesting such information. Instead, over ensuing decades, costs increased incrementally and became more complex, and institutions paid their unrecovered indirect cost dollars out of multiple budgets, most of which were not even predominantly devoted to maintaining research. No one (federal, private, or in the institution itself) bothered to ask where any of the money for indirect costs "really" came from. Also, it became clear that even superb documentation of unrecovered indirect costs (e.g., UCSF's \$164M in FY2014) would never affect an outcome of "negotiation" with a federal agency. Thus, incrementally, the M-UP has rendered unrecovered indirect costs—however large—essentially unknowable.

Finally, we have described many ways in which the federal government limits its quantitative obligation to pay ICR, but that does not mean that we think the government should pay all the indirect costs of research. Like other research universities, UCSF at present pays a substantial portion of those indirect costs (Fig. 3-3); this is as it should be,, because the institution derives great benefits from the research it produces, which attracts faculty, students, patients, and philanthropic donors, and furnishes the immense satisfaction that comes from advancing knowledge and medical care. For all academic research institutions, however, indirect costs pose two extremely difficult questions.

1. How should the relative portions of indirect costs paid by funding agencies vs. the institution be determined? The present system is both cumbersome and potentially unfair with respect to certain types of research and some universities. These problems reflect a long, complex

political history and cannot be fixed without extensive reform of the present rules and regulations—a daunting task indeed!

2. Where are universities to find the money to pay their share of indirect costs? For rich private research universities, the answer is philanthropy. For public universities like UCSF, the answer is by no means clear. Sharp reductions in state support make it hard for all state universities to pay for their research programs. For a biomedical institution like UCSF, tuition can contribute very little, and philanthropy is much harder to obtain than for private universities with many rich alumni. UCSF can leverage some of its clinical income toward research, but this resource is also limited.

We cannot provide satisfying answers to either of these thorny questions, but later chapters will make it clear that both questions have implications for the future of academic research in general, and UCSF's research, in particular.

Chapter 4

Money is a good soldier: Buildings, equity, gifts, and debt

Until now our account of UCSF's finances has focused on revenues, with occasional nods toward expenditures. Now we begin to explore how the institution manages to leverage its assets to meet its aspirations. This chapter sets the stage by discussing three critical topics. First we describe UCSF's "real" assets—its buildings and space devoted to various missions in different locations. Second, we outline rudiments of how the institution forecasts the future and plans accordingly. Finally, we consider how UCSF leverages its assets by spending cash (or equity), seeking state funding (on ever-rarer occasions), seeking philanthropic gifts, or borrowing funds for buildings or projects.

Buildings and Space

To fulfill all its missions, UCSF needs durable, well-designed physical spaces. Such spaces are classified under four main functional categories: teaching (also termed "Instructional"), research, clinical care, and support. *Teaching* space is devoted to educating professional students, graduate students, clinicians in training, etc.; it includes not only classrooms and lecture halls, but also faculty offices, space dedicated to educational support staff, conferences, and study space. The search for new knowledge takes place in *research* space: "wet-bench" laboratories, research equipment rooms, dry-lab offices for computation and analysis, and related support spaces. Patients are seen and treated in *clinical care* space: hospital rooms for sick patients, emergency room facilities, operating rooms, treatment rooms, nursing stations, waiting rooms, and any type of room that directly supports clinical care of in-patients or out-patients. *Support space* is all the other space necessary to support performance of those three primary missions, including libraries, parking garages, food service facili-

**Table 4-1. Research Space *vs.* Total Space
at Different Sites***

Campus	Total space		Research Space[¶]		
	asf[§]	% of total	asf	% at site	% all UCSF research
Fresno	58,616	1.0	0	0	0.0
Mission Bay	1,641,647	29	621,219	38	43
Mt Zion	532,403	9.3	66,817	13	4.7
Parnassus	2,138,222	33	514,090	24	36
SFGH[§]	246,047	4.4	95,203	39	6.6
Other sites[†]	1,106,169	19	132,528	12	9.3
Total	5,723,604	100	1,430,857	25	100

*Data in this table was from reference *2*.
†Other sites include: Several, including Laurel Heights, China Basin, and Mission Center.
¶Research space includes laboratories, research offices, and miscellaneous.
§Abbreviations: asf, assignable square feet (*1*); SFGH, San Francisco General Hospital.

ties, and spaces for administration, police and security, computer services, etc.

Different spaces in any particular building may fall into one, several, or all four categories, and two or even three missions may take place in a single space or room. Teaching often takes place, for instance, in research labs, clinical examining rooms, and patients' sick-rooms, and patient-focused research can take place in space otherwise devoted to clinical care. While inevitably overlapping functions sometimes confuse, the University of California and higher education throughout the US try to make sure that a particular space's major function defines its primary use.

UCSF's total space, distributed among multiple sites (Table 4-1), amounts to 5.7 million assignable square feet (asf)—a measure roughly equivalent to "usable" square feet (*1*). Of these sites, two account for 62% of the total: the Parnassus campus (33%) and the Mission Bay campus (29%). Of UCSF's total space, 1.43 million asf (26%) are devoted to research (Tables 4-1 and 4-2; *2*). Of UCSF's total research space, 79% is located on the two largest campuses—36% at Parnassus and 43% at the Mission Bay campus (Table 4-1). Table 4-2 compares space devoted to research (including laboratories, research offices, and research support facilities) vs. that devoted to other uses, UCSF-wide. Counting all UCSF campuses, more asf are devoted to administrative offices than to research (28 and 25% of total UCSF space, respectively), but the asf devoted to each of these two uses far surpasses any other uses, including clinical care (14%).

Table 4-2. Space for Research and Other Uses (UCSF-wide)*

Use of Space	asf§	%
Acad§ office	280,860	4.9
Clinic	822,780	14
Conference	179,857	3.1
Housing	484,878	8.5
Instruc§	99,247	1.7
Office (administration)	1,578,010	28
Other uses†	847,115	15
Research	1,430,857	25
Total	5,723,604	100

*Data in this table is from reference 2. Reference 2 was not updated with the final space information for the new UCSF Hospital at Mission Bay at the time of publication.
†Other uses are multiple; among the largest are storage, animal quarters, food faciltiies and service.
§Abbreviations: asf, assignable square feet, Acad, Academic; Instruc, Instructional

Academic biomedical researchers need space to do their research, and institutions badly need every dollar of the indirect costs they recover when research dollars are spent. In earlier years, PIs urged their institutions to provide more laboratory space, so they could expand their research programs with dollars readily obtained from NIH. In contrast, now many researchers complain that they are constantly pushed to obtain more grant dollars by host institutions dependent on indirect cost recovery (ICR). This ICR is surely critical, for UCSF and most other research institutions. How do institutions maintain or increase the ICR flow?

UCSF's interest in ICR is serious, and not only because ICR is needed to maintain research. Indeed, the Chancellor's UCSF Space Committee uses ICR as a general indicator of the relative magnitude and intensity of research in planning for new buildings or changes in the function of existing buildings. In 2010, the Space Committee began to use ICR as an explicit criterion for judging whether research space is efficiently utilized, based on the following stated policy (3): "For appropriate spaces (e.g., Research) a standard expected level of extramural funding (indirect costs; $/asf) will be defined for such space based on operational costs. . . . Failure to meet the overall expected level of funding for a Unit is one criterion that could support a Space Committee recommendation to decrease the total asf assigned to the Unit. [A]ll units will be expected to demonstrate extramural Facilities and Administration (F&A) recovery in excess of $90 per asf. . . . The [UCSF Space] Committee will re-assess this figure on an annual basis. . . . [If s]pace is deemed to not be used efficiently . . . , this space will be returned to the Chancellor." In January 2016, the criterion will increase from $90/asf to $120/asf (4). In principle, then, every unit's research asf will depend quantitatively upon its faculty's ability to maintain ICR on their grant awards at or above a specified level. The criterion applies to average ICR dollars per asf in all academic units (schools, depart-ments, ORUs, etc.), but does not specify that each of the unit's individual faculty laboratories must meet the criterion.

Some faculty members bridle at being assessed to furnish ICR as surro-gate rent for the privilege of directing a research program, but it is hard to see how UCSF can avoid setting some kind of standard, because its research en-terprise depends on ICR (and on direct costs as well) to survive in the face of progressive loss of state financial support, fierce competition for researchers, students, and grant dollars, and ever-increasing costs constructing laboratories and conducting and administering research.

Nonetheless, the ICR/asf policy itself appears to us as counterproduc-tive, standing by itself. The problem is not only that unthinking state and federal politicians may use the notion of ICR as surrogate rent as a red flag to promote anti-research and anti-academic agendas. More important, in choos-ing ICR/asf as *the* quantitative criterion for utilization of research space, UCSF is adopting a dangerously blunt instrument for the delicate, crucial task of assessing *the value of a research project* in relation to the space it uses, for four reasons:

1. ICR on federal projects is determined by arcane, arbitrary rules (chapter 3) that bear no relation to the value of those research projects.
2. Different kinds of research earn ICR at very different rates in relation to space utilized (e.g., dry-lab vs. wet-lab research, as we shall see in chapters 7-9).
3. Because ICR is much lower for privately than for federally funded research (chapter 3), projects can earn more (or less) ICR for reasons unrelated to research quality.
4. Because research support from the Howard Hughes Medical Institute (HHMI) pays no ICR whatever, any unit that houses HHMI investigators will report lower ICR/asf.

Even as a benchmark for the relative density of research in a particular building or space, the quantitative criterion should surely include both direct and indirect costs, simply because the university clearly needs both. Also, for the University to decide whether an academic unit should gain or lose research space, it must explicitly judge the *quality* of the research it conducts, because that quality determines the worth of research to the university and society as a whole. (High UCSF officials told the authors that the ICR benchmark is only one of eight criteria used for judging utilization of research space, but we were not able to find the other seven criteria in the policy statement (*3*) that announces the use of ICR dollars per asf as the key quantitative criterion.) To judge quality requires answering this question: does new knowledge produced by this research increase our understanding of the natural world and/or our ability to understand and treat disease? While large institutions naturally seek simple numerical answers to hard questions, the ICR/asf criterion can produce *wrong* answers (see above). Correct answers can and should depend on judgments by the best impartial scientists the institution itself can find in its faculty and assign to this task—not to those whose expertise limits them to measuring only asf and ICR. Arbitrary dependence on numbers did not make UCSF a first-rate research institution. Instead, research quality requires careful value judgments—not hasty shortcuts.

A Short History: How UCSF Pays for its Research Facilities

To prepare for more extensive discussion of how UCSF now pays for its research facilities, we begin by asking where the money came from in the 20th century (*5*). Before about 1980, the state of California paid most of the bills for UCSF's new facilities, including hospitals; other bills—for teaching, research, administrative, and support facilities—were also paid by the state, with minor contributions from philanthropic donors. Then and now, funds for housing, food service, and parking facilities were paid from debt supported by revenues earned from these services. Later, the state paid less than half the bill for constructing Long Hospital, completed in the 1980s; by the mid-1990s, the state virtually stopped funding UCSF's hospital construction and renovation. From then on, state support for UCSF research facilities has been virtually nil, owing in part to the recession of 1991-94, the "dot.com" crash of 2001-03, the 2008 real-estate crash, and the subsequent recession. For two decades, the state has funded UC teaching facilities, almost exclusively; almost no teaching facility dollars came to UCSF.

To become acquainted with the different mechanisms by which UCSF pays for its facilities, consider capital funding of the $1.586B Mission Bay

Table 4-3. Mission Bay Capital Funding Plan*

	Gifts $M†	Campus Debt $M	Garamendi Debt $M	Housing Debt $M	Parking Debt $M	Capital Lease $M	Campus Reserves $M	State $M	Total $M
Genentech Hall	110.0	70.0					14.0	21.0	215.0
Byers Hall			40.0					55.0	95.0
Rock Hall	48.0						41.4		89.4
Rutter Center	60.0						9.6		69.6
Diller Cancer Res.†	91.4	30.0					21.0		142.4
Housing Block 20	9.0			103.0			4.1		116.1
Parking					39.0		2.5		41.5
Central Utility Plant		18.0					5.5		23.5
CVRI Building	31.0	209					14.0		254.0
Sandler Neurosci.†						208.0			208.0
Mission Hall	20.0	84.4					14.2		118.6
Diller 4th Floor							17.9		17.9
Blocks 33/34 Acqu.		108.6							108.6
Infrastructure	12.0	37.0					37.0		86.0
Total $M	381.4	557.0	40.0	103.0	39.0	208.0	181.2	76.0	1,585.6
%	24.1	35.1	2.5	6.5	2.5	13.1	11.4	4.8	100

*Data in this table is from reference 6.
†Abbreviations: Acqu., Acquisition; CVRI, Cardiovascular Research Institute; Neurosci., Neurosciences Building; Res., Research Building; $M, millions of dollars.

campus, building by building (Table 4-3), and money sources for each (Table 4-4); the tables are based on a capital funding plan that began in 1997, and was updated in 2015 (6). Most Mission Bay construction is funded from more than a single source (Table 4-3), often including philanthropic gifts, campus reserves, and one of several "flavors" of debt (described more fully below). Note also the exception to our statement that state support for UCSF's research construction has been "virtually nil" for decades: the state of California paid $76M—i.e., only 4.8% ($76M) of all Mission Bay construction, as we saw earlier (7).

Table 4-4 summarizes the four distinct mechanisms used to pay for these projects. Philanthropic *gifts* are paying 24% of the new campus's construction costs. The second mechanism, ordinary debt ($739M), pays for 47%. Principal and interest on this debt comes from three different sources of campus income: ICR backs most of it ($597M), with income from housing and parking services paying off the corresponding auxiliary debts. The third mechanism, *operating or capital leases*, represent a different flavor of debt, explained later in this chapter; this source accounts for 14% of the new campus's cost. The final source is *equity*—basically cash, which UCSF obtains either from cash reserves (11% of the new campus's costs) or state funds (4.8%). The next section describes details of these modes of payment and rules that govern them.

**Table 4-4. Mission Bay Capital
Funding: Payment Summary***

Mode of payment	Cost	
	M	% Total
Gifts	381	24
Debt	739	47
ICR[†§]	*597*	*38*
Housing income[†]	*103*	*6.5*
Parking income[†]	*39*	*2.5*
Capital Lease	208	14
Equity	181	11
State	76	4.8
Total	1,586	100

*Data in the table is from ref. *6*.
†Items in italics are subsets of the sources for payment of the debt ($739M) listed in the line above; the dollar figures are for the individual items, while the corresponding percentage figures refer to percentages of total payment sources in the table.
§Abbreviations: ICR, indirect cost recovery; $M, millions of dollars

Leveraging Assets for the Future

UCSF is an educational institution that must also operate as a business to compete effectively for patients and dollars against other health care enterprises, and also against large, academically strong, well-funded research institutions that vie against one another to maintain—and often to increase—the number and quality of their researchers, students, and sponsored research funds. Like any dynamic business, UCSF husbands and increases its resources by predicting and planning for the future. To do so, it maintains a Core Financial Plan (CFP) and forecasting effort that combine its financial plans for the clinical enterprise (UCSF Health) and for the central resources controlled by its Schools and Chancellor's Office. In autumn each year, the CFP assesses the past fiscal year and forecasts revenues and expenses for the next decade.

Such forecasts incorporate detailed inferences and assumptions with respect to operating costs and growth, extant debt payments, and new capital projects for new construction and maintenance or upgrading of present facilities. Based on past performance and prudent assumptions about changes in the economic environment, forecasts help leaders make hard decisions. Do we pay for X with cash reserves or by borrowing? How much philanthropy can project X attract? Can we backstop shortfalls in philanthropy, if they occur? To cover unanticipated problems with X, how many dollars should be set aside? (What about projects Y, Z, M, N, and P?) Incorporating best guesses and calculations for ongoing operations and future projects, forecasters predict bottom lines for subsequent years. If revenues from project X exceed its costs, the institution gains "resources on the margin," which businesses call "profit." A non-profit enterprise, UCSF uses resources on the margin to meet future goals, satisfy requirements and regulations (e.g., earthquake safety), and fulfill compelling aspirations.

This section now turns its attention to the different sources of funds—equity and public funding, philanthropic gifts, and various forms of debt—used by UCSF to create new space, replace old space, or renovate existing space to make it functional in future years. The actual decision-making process will be described in chapter 5.

Equity, including public funds. Equity is simply "available cash," in the form of current funds or reserves. The decision to use such money is often dictated by exigent need or unforeseen circumstances, conditions that account for much of the campus reserves UCSF has spent to maintain construction of the Mission Bay campus, amounting so far to $181M, of about 11% of the project's total cost (Table 4-2).

In addition to available cash, UCSF has in the past treated public funding as a form of equity, despite the fact that state funding is usually provided by general obligation bonds, repaid from state tax revenues. Such state funds—sweet, but hard to get—may entail three-year delays between initial request and receipt of actual funds—time devoted to internal review by UC, further review by a state agency, and a political process that can attach strings to each dollar. During the past 15 years, UCSF obtained funds via this route for two projects related to its education mission (*8*). Sometimes, small windfalls occur for research buildings, as with the special state bond funds that paid $55M of the $95M cost of constructing Byers Hall (aka the California Institute for Science and Innovation) or a seismic code replacement project that helped to pay $21M of the $215M cost for Genentech Hall (Table 4-3). For 35 years, UCSF has attracted no federal construction grants; federal dollars for higher education buildings are rare.

Philanthropy. Dollars from generous donors are almost always welcome. A donor may attach onerous demands or stipulations to a gift, but most gifts—whoever the donor may be—come with two kinds of unavoidable costs:

1. As we noted in chapter 2, donors may pledge contributions over a period of years, so the university incurs a cost for paying interest charges

to accept the gift. Paid over 10 years, a gift of $100M could cost the university over $20M in interest costs (e.g., with a bridge loan for 10 years at 5% interest).

2. A major fund-raising campaign can cost up to $3-5M per year for a campaign that requires additional fund-raisers and support staff, sponsors fund-raising events, and it can last for five years. Skilled fund-raisers receive premium pay because they are engaged for short times, and in San Francisco living costs drive their salaries higher.

For these reasons, raising $350M for new research facilities over a five-year period could cost a university $75M or more in operating costs plus interest costs for unpaid gift pledges. UCSF's initial donation target to build the Mission Bay campus was $350M, and its first phase raised $329M. We do not know how much it cost to raise that money. The present total, $381M (Table 4-3), represents one of every four dollars used to build the campus so far. Now a specific target is usually set for each new building.

Debt. For major research universities, debt is an essential tool for building and renewing teaching and research facilities. Private universities have used debt and gifts for many decades, because they can repay their debts from several sources, including income from tuition, general endowment, and other investments. Unable to secure loans in such ways, public institutions arrived late at the banquet, because their general endowments are meager and states generally prohibit use of tuition to repay debt. Fortunately, by the late 1980s, UCSF (and other public research universities) finally began to use ICR on federal and private contracts and grants as a pledge-able revenue, vetted by Wall Street bankers and debt-rating agencies, for securing (and paying) debt. UCSF didn't know at that the time that this use of ICR would prove critical for its survival during the ensuing 25 "lean" years, which simultaneously increased the need for borrowed money and made it impossible to rely on steady state support.

Before 1986, UCSF issued only small amounts of debt, for parking facilities and some student housing. In that year the institution issued its first ICR-backed debt, when it borrowed $55M to purchase and update the Laurel Heights facility in San Francisco. Thirty years later, its present debt comes to $2.0B, comprising $900 million for the clinical enterprise and $1.1B for the Campus, which included $162M for auxiliary enterprises like parking and housing, for which both interest and repayment of the principal are paid from the income of each separate enterprise (*9*).

Now UCSF's debt pays for a wide range of capital programs. On the

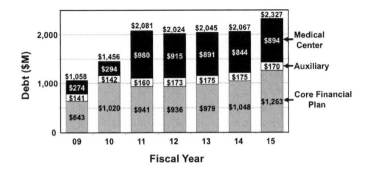

Fig. 4-1. UCSF debt doubled between FY2009 and 2015 (*9*). Each column shows the institution's debt in a particular fiscal year (abscissa); the debt is apportioned in three segments, shown from top to bottom: the clinical enterprise (Medical Center); auxiliary (to be paid by income from auxiliary functions for which the debt is incurred); academic campus (aka the Chancellor's Core Financial Plan).

Parnassus campus these include renewal and seismic upgrading of older buildings, replacement of heating, power plant, utility systems, and creation of a new animal care facilities and the Dolby Regeneration Medicine building. In other locations, debt allowed acquisition of facilities at Mission Center, a new medical education center in Fresno, and the Osher Center at Mount Zion. Development of the $1.586B new research campus at Mission Bay has relied heavily on debt (Table 4-3), as described above. Proportionately, debt so far is paying 47% of the total cost, with a capital lease (a specialized form of debt) accounting for an additional 13%; gifts, campus reserves, and the state of California account, respectively, for 24, 11, and 4.8% of the total (Table 4-4).

Capital or operating leases are names for arrangements very like ordinary debt. In these leases, the final product is "bought" by annual payments that require continuing sources of available funds—a requirement identical to that used in normally issued debt. For example, UCSF purchased the Sandler Neuroscience Research Building (Table 4-3) via a capital lease, based on "a ground lease-development-leaseback" scenario. In simpler terms, the institution owns the land, contracts with an outside party to develop a project as specified by the owner, and pays the developer back through a lease arrangement. In such a "capital lease," the owner (UCSF) takes over the project when the development period ends (in this case, after 30 years). (In a so-called "operating" lease, the institution pays over time but does not intend to own the project at the end.)

During the six years between FY2009 and FY2015, UCSF's total debt more than doubled, rising from about $1.06B to $2.33B (Fig. 4-1; *9*). Overall,

Table 4-5. Additional Planned UCSF Debt, FY2015-FY2025*

Project	Financing Year	Debt ($M)[†]
Core Financial Plan[†]		
Renovations at Parnassus & SFGH[§]	2015-2024	391
MB[§] Block 23A Building	2018-19	161
Block 33/34 Bldg[§]	2018-19	159
Subtotal, Core Financial Plan		711
Auxiliaries[†]		
Mission Bay Surface Parking	2016	8
Mission Bay Housing	2019	221
UC Hall Seismic Refit (Housing)	2019	32
Proctor Building Demolition	2017-18	2
MU/ACC[§] Garage Spall Repair PH2	2019	17
Subtotal, Auxiliaries		280
Total		991

*Data in the table is from reference 9.

†The Core Financial Plan (CFP) and Auxiliaries are two separate categories of debt: the CFP debt is paid by the campus (supervised by the Chancellor's Office), from equity and philanthropy, while auxiliary debts are paid from revenues of the campus's auxiliary functions, such as parking, housing, etc.

§Abbreviations: Bldg, Building; MB, Mission Bay; MSB, Medical Sciences Building (Parnassus campus); MU/ACC, Millberry Union/Acute Care Center (Parnassus campus); SFGH, San Francisco General Hospital; $M, millions of dollars.

the FY2014 debt was 1.95-fold that carried by UCSF in FY2009. Most of that change reflected a 3.08-fold change (that is, a 208% increase) in debt incurred by the clinical enterprise ("Medical Center" in Figs. 4-1, 4-2, and 4-3), owing primarily to constructing new hospital facilities at Mission Bay. Debt carried by the academic campus (called the "Core Financial Plan" in these figures) rose less (by ~63%) over this period, again predominantly due to obligations incurred for Mission Bay construction. Debt on auxiliary functions like parking and housing rose even less (by 24%).

Predicting Future Debt

Because future debt obligations inevitably constrain future options and opportunities, large institutions carefully plan how to distribute future issuances of debt. In December 2015, UCSF's planners expected the university to incur new debts over the coming decade (Table 4-5), {Table 4-5 here} based on capital the university would borrow at specific times (9). These planning numbers are subject to change, of course, but they reveal UCSF's thinking about its plans for the coming 10-year time window. As we write, some items on the

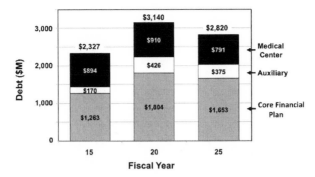

Fig. 4-2. UCSF debt will increase from about $2.1B in FY2014 to $2.5B in FY2024 (9). The debt (correct for 2014, predicted for the two other fiscal years) is apportioned in the same categories described in the Fig. 4-1 legend.

list have already been initiated.

If each project is financed at the amount shown in Table 4-5, by FY2026 UCSF's debt level will increase from the 2015 figure (~$2.33B) to ~$2.82B (Fig. 4-2; 9). Issuing those planned new debts means UCSF will require more cash in future to meet its debt obligations—i.e., to "service" that debt over the long term—as indicated in Fig. 4-3 (9): annual costs of debt service are projected to more than double, from ~$102M in FY2015 to ~$231M in FY2025. After an additional 24 years, in FY2049, annual debt service would fall back down to a value close to that of FY2015—providing that UCSF issues no further debt in the interim. "No further debt," of course, is an untenable as-

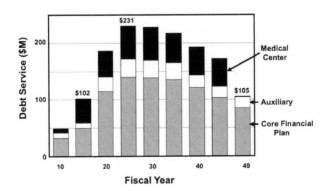

Fig. 4-3. Annual debt service (payment of principal and interest) is predicted to double between FY15 and FY25 (9). Here debt service is apportioned in the same categories shown for debt in Figs. 4-1 and 4-2. If UCSF were to incur no further debt since 2015, debt service would decline after FY2025, but that fall is in fact unlikely, owing to debt that will be issued in future years, as explained in the main text.

sumption; although the prediction shows debt service costs if UCSF incurs no further debt than that explicitly planned in 2015, additional debts will certainly be issued during the coming 34 years. For instance, by 2024 some Mission Bay buildings, nearly 25 years old, will need renewal and upgrades. And UCSF's Long Range Development Plan (*10*), which looks forward to 2035, discusses additional needs, soon to appear on the planning horizon.

Finally, it is worth pointing out the bold optimism that underlies planning for future debt levels: such plans assume that medical care continues to thrive as a profitable business and that steady streams of federal dollars continue to flow in support of both patient care and biomedical research. For biomedical research, the latter assumption has not been valid for more than a decade (see chapter 7, below); neither it nor the other assumptions are assured over the longer term. Chapters 5 and 10 will return to these issues.

Priorities and Decision Making: Faith vs. Risk

In 2010, Bruce Alberts warned that the combination of soft-money salaries and ICR from the NIH to reimburse interest and depreciation on research buildings "enables the many advocates for expansion [of academic research institutions] to effectively argue that the costs will eventually be borne in large part by the U.S. government" (*11*). As we shall see, this statement does not correctly describe an institution's decision to build a specific research building. It *does* apply, however, to long-term expansion of UCSF and other research institutions. As described above, UCSF uses the reliability of its ICR income to show prospective lenders that their loans will be paid. Approximately 25% (~$45M) of that ICR income in 2014 (*12*) was reimbursement for interest and depreciation of research facilities built in previous decades. Thus institutional expansion rests squarely on faith that federal support for research will continue. Later we shall return to this faith, and the genuine risks it poses for the institution and its lenders.

First, however, consider short-term decisions for building a specific research facility. Reliance on future ICR played little if any role in such decisions at UCSF, as shown by direct observation of the decision process from 1991 to 2013 (*13*). Back when state taxes paid for most research facilities, UCSF could enjoy the fruits of new construction without worrying much about either costs or using ICR to pay them. In the early 1990s, however, UC began sharply to reduce its support for construction of research facilities. As a result, the institution learned a new lesson: *over the short term, every research facility is a losing proposition*, because it incurs costs much higher than the ICR it earns.

In 1990, a new state law (*14*) allowed UC to finance construction of new research facilities by using 100% of net new ICR generated from support for research in the new buildings. At the time, and for some years thereafter, more than 50% of all ICR went not to the campuses where the sponsored research was conducted, but was instead divided by the state of California and UC's central administration (see Fig. 3-1). For this reason UCSF and other campuses greeted the new "Garamendi financing mechanism" (14) with enormous enthusiasm, because now they would retain all the ICR earned by research in new laboratories built by Garamendi loans (*15*).

Naturally, there was a catch: UCSF (like other UC campuses) also had to operate and maintain such buildings from the same new ICR revenue, or from any excess dollars it might scrape together. UCSF used the new mechanism to construct a new cancer research building at its Mt. Zion campus. The Garamendi financing mechanism permitted UCSF to accumulate a financial deficit on operating and debt costs while the new facility filled with faculty investigators and new research grants; the accumulated deficit was then to be paid back from ICR in excess of the new building's annual operating, maintenance and debt payment costs. Applying the Garamendi mechanism to pay for the new cancer building soon produced serious problems:

1. It quickly became clear that that years would pass before the new facility realized its full potential as a magnet for ICR—at least three years for planning and constructing the building, plus an unknown number of years to find, attract, and relocate research faculty able to develop exciting new research programs and populate the new laboratories. (Otherwise, the new faculty and staff would have to be housed in some kind of holding center if they were to enter the building when it opened.) How long would that be? On what basis was the new ICR going to be projected?

2. A net increase in research faculty, staff, and equipment inevitably creates a need for more administration (e.g., for payroll, grants, etc.), which accounted for more than 50% of total ICR in the early 1990s. Where could UCSF find the money to pay administrators when the Garamendi mechanism required it to use 100% of ICR generated by the new research for maintenance, utilities, and interest costs?

3. What would happen if the new research program theme fizzled and the building's research generated ICR at only pennies on the dollar? Who would pay the bills?

Fortunately, but also very slowly, scary risks became happy results. Five years after its opening, the building had been occupied by enough new investigators to generate net new research dollars, with help from its research program being named as one of a very few national cancer centers; it took three additional years for those researchers' new grants to generate enough ICR to begin paying all the building's utility, operating, and maintenance costs, as well as the debt payments; five *more* years were necessary for the ICR to pay off the operating and administrative deficits generated in the previous eight years. So, after a delay of 13 years, ICR dollars earned by research in the building were finally able to pay for the ongoing costs and administrative support needed to build, staff, and maintain the new facility. Ultimately, 100% of the ICR paid the bills, but the mechanism hardly constituted a viable business model for generating future revenue. The take-home message: over the near term, it is folly to rely on generating excess ICR income as the primary driver for constructing research facilities.

As we suggested earlier, there is a bigger issue. Stated most broadly, research universities are driven by hope and exciting opportunities, but repeatedly encounter unpredictable realities. Stated a different way, the issue involves not only judging short-term risks, but also not falling into the fatal trap of taking the longer term for granted. UCSF appears to have judged short-term risks pretty accurately, and has profited from a six-decade run of extraordinary luck. But can its research mission be sustained, long term? Will funding sources of research universities remain viable? As we saw in earlier chapters, trust in government research funding is an act of faith. State governments in general, and that of California in particular, have not proved reliable partners. Over the past decade, flat-lined NIH budgets show that unquestioned reliance on the federal government is also short-sighted. The same, often, is true for philanthropy. Each source is exquisitely susceptible to rapid changes and uncertainties, political, social, and economic. Will health sciences research find a reliable and sustainable funding model for its future?

We return to these questions in chapters 5 and 10.

Chapter 5

Sweet uses of adversity: Planning for change

As they try to distribute resources wisely, UCSF and other large academic research institutions repeatedly face hard decisions about how to change that distribution in the face of new opportunities and challenges. To coordinate agile, correct decisions, UCSF has had to develop ways to analyze its resources and make long-range plans. This chapter describes how, since the 1960s, UCSF's responses to its own success and to external dangers triggered successive changes in planning, decision making, and distribution of responsibility for making and coordinating those decisions. The chapter concludes by highlighting key aspects of the latest (2015) version of UCSF's 10-year financial plan (1)—aspects which will, in turn, prove critical for understanding our proposals for changing the future of biomedical research at UCSF, in chapter 10.

Parnassus Will Not Suffice: Long-range Development Plans (LRDPs), 1962-1995

We begin our history with a long view, depicted in a series of LRDPs for UCSF, from 1962 to 2015. The LRDP of 1962 revealed ambitious plans for expanding facilities and projects in and around the Parnassus campus, including projected growth south of the campus, on Mt. Sutro, and the Inner Sunset neighborhood. Opposition to expansion by neighborhood activists, however, led to a second LRDP (1976), which revised and curtailed expansion plans. Later that year, UCSF also agreed to fix the Parnassus site's geographic boundaries and accept a ceiling on the site's total square feet of developed space.

Those limitations soon conflicted directly with the beginning of UCSF's increasing success, both as a center for human health research and also—with the development of DNA technology and discovery of oncogenes—as a world leader in basic science research. With lightning speed (in academia six years is fast), yet another LRDP (1982) gained UCSF some breathing time, as an agreement with neighborhood groups allowed UCSF to exceed modestly the space "ceiling" of 1976 and build a new library and small research buildings, in return for promising to demolish several old "temporary" buildings.

The 1982 LRDP's bottom line was a gob-smacker: unable to grow at the Parnassus site, UCSF would develop satellite sites in and near San Francisco. At first, activities not directly required for teaching, research, or patient care were moved away from the Parnassus campus—"de-centralized," in LRDP parlance—to satellite campuses, including Laurel Heights and Mission Center, each with more than 300,000 square feet. Some functions were moved to affiliated campuses like San Francisco General Medical Center and the VA Medical Center; at both sites, where UCSF participates in staffing, management, and operations, and also trains its students. Also, UCSF acquired an additional medical center campus, now called the UCSF Mt. Zion Medical Center.

Soon these sites were over-crowded with decentralized operations and expanding research and clinical programs. Although UCSF appeared remarkably efficient in accomplishing much in little space, decentralizing support functions and distributing a few research programs to separate physical locations treated the symptoms, but could not fix the central problem. By 1989, a UCSF Faculty Futures Committee, appointed by the Chancellor, concluded that continued restriction on growth at Parnassus would require UCSF to build or acquire an additional major campus.

A New Site at Mission Bay

As the institution's best of times alternated with its worst, both shaped hopes and plans for its future, and gradually fashioned a model for planning resources and making long-term decisions. In a key first step, yet another LRDP (1996) defined a second primary site should look like, what programs it should house, and how it should relate to existing campuses. This LRDP opened doors not only to a new research campus, but also to: (i) expanding the clinical mission, with a new hospital and medical offices, to replace seismically-deficient facilities at Parnassus; (ii) accommodating more students and medical residents in housing owned and operated by UCSF; (iii) providing "campus life services" to students, faculty, staff and the neighboring community.

A year later, in 1997, UCSF accepted an immensely valuable gift: the Mission Bay campus on the eastern edge of San Francisco, a few miles from Parnassus. (The site's joint donors: the city of San Francisco and the Mission Bay site developer, Catellus Corporation.) Since then, UCSF has spent nearly $1.6B on its new research campus, plus student housing, parking structures, and a major recreation and conference facility as well (*2*). With an additional ~$1.5B, it acquired adjacent property and has built a new Women and Children's hospital and an adult cancer hospital with attendant supporting clinics, medical office buildings and parking facilities (*3*). In 2014, UCSF published a new LRDP (*4*), focused on plans for its teaching, research and clinical care missions up to 2035.

The Resource Planning Evolution

In the half century since the 1962 LRDP, UCSF transformed itself from an institution with a single site, a simple mission, and about 10,000 employees into a leading health center that produces new understanding of biology and pathogenesis, new treatments for human disease, and highly skilled medical professionals and research scientists. Its nearly 30,000 employees and students are located at five major sites in San Francisco and dozens of others in the Bay area and northern and central California. How did its ability to plan future resources and make long-range decisions change to enable this extraordinary growth and metamorphosis?

Early on, UCSF seemed to receive almost all its funds from the state of California—for employee salaries, construction of buildings, and just about everything else. But this impression was wrong: in FY1979, only ~27% of UCSF's revenues came from the state, with 25% from federal government, 28% from its hospitals, 10% from its clinical practice income, and 10% from other sources (*5*). Still, state funds were the primary focus of financial planning, for both UC and UCSF. Minutes of UC Regents' meetings in the fall of each year, focused on the UC budget plan, were devoted almost entirely to state funds. The State Educational Appropriation (SEA) was less than 4% of UCSF's budget in FY2014 (chapter 1), much less than in earlier days: for instance, in FY1971 UCSF's SEA was ~48% of its total budget and SEAs at general UC campuses like Berkeley, Los Angeles, Davis, and San Diego were even higher (~64-74%; *6*).

At every administrative level, resource planning in earlier days was largely confined to state funds. UC left to UCSF responsibility for managing revenues of UCSF's medical center (and physician fees), and UCSF's chancellor left that responsibility pretty much to the Medical Center director and the Medical School Dean. So UCSF's planning model was born "decentralized," although the buzzword was not much used in 1970.

Impact of Indirect Cost Recovery (ICR) on Resource Planning

As NIH-funded research grew across the US and at several UC campuses, so did ICR. Beginning in the 1960s, UC campuses were required to deliver any ICR they earned back to the UC President's Office, with no substantive return to the campuses. Finally, in FY1983, UC President David Saxon grudgingly responded to a publicity crisis stirred by several UC campuses, including UCSF (7), by returning part of their ICR back to the campuses. Up until that point (and thereafter, as well) a portion of the ICR had been used to "subvent" the SEA (readers should always view the word, "subvent," as a hint of possible deception; 8) with the rest of the ICR held by the President to dole out for special purposes. (Special purposes included helping to pay costs for developing the small new campuses at Santa Cruz and Irvine, and expansion of older campuses at Santa Barbara and Riverside—including in most cases construction costs the state chose not to fund from its own coffers.) The President's Office made no effort to relate the amount of ICR doled out in relation to who earned it. So, UCSF and UC San Diego (which at the time, like UCSF, had relatively few undergraduate students) had to pony up tens of millions of dollars each year, receiving no evident benefit in return.

The President's FY1983 decision to return part of their ICR to the campuses still failed to satisfy UCSF. Instead of returning all the ICR not needed to subvent state funds in proportion to where it was generated, the President's Office devised a clever formula, which gave UCSF about 45 cents on its ICR dollar (9). While finally receiving part of its ICR was better than a sharp stick in the eye, the allocation formula caused friction for 18 more years, when Richard Atkinson, then University President, allocated 96% of all ICR earned each year to the campuses that earned it.

Nonetheless, in 1983 UCSF's Chancellor finally did receive a small proportion of UCSF's ICR—unrestricted dollars, substantial enough to make something happen. An early result: the Chancellor created a new position, Vice Chancellor for Resource Management and Planning (VC-RMP), with the goal of making resource planning and financial management play key strategic roles in UCSF's future development. (Later called Vice Chancellor—Finance, this position is now called Associate Vice Chancellor—Budget & Resource Management.) Creation of the new position coincided—probably not fortuitously—with growing awareness that UCSF would not expand further at Parnassus, so the new VC-RMP was needed to coordinate development at other sites.

As one of his first tasks, this VC-RMP, Tom Rolinson, initiated an effort to raise the ICR rate UCSF earned on federal grants from its then piddling rate of 27.7% to a rate closer to the ~80% rate then earned by other leading research universities (*10*). He set up a cost accounting system and hired and trained professional staff, so that federal auditors soon gave UCSF the maximum allowable increase at each successive rate negotiation (for details of this one-sided negotiation, see chapter 3). During the next three decades the first allocation of a few million dollars has grown to almost $200M per year, providing most of the Chancellor's Campus Core Funds (CCF; *11*). To acquire UCSF's first two major satellites, the Laurel Heights and Mission Center campuses, the Chancellor used debt backed by ICR for the acquisitions, and ICR to pay for their operations.

Despite the new VC-RMP position, no formal planning or strategy model was put into place for the next 10 years. During these "black box model" years, the VC-RMP's staff did initiate a comprehensive framework for organizing the Chancellor's funds (largely State funds, a few endowments and the new ICR allocation), but referred to it simply as a "checkbook," because it functioned mainly as a mechanism for recording decisions, rather than as a tool for planning or making decisions. Later (1986-1990), the VC-RMP worked to establish firm annual budgets for at least the Chancellor's administration and the CCF, with annual review of resource needs, future plans, and pending regulatory requirements that might require outlays of funds. But back doors into offices of the Chancellor or the Senior Vice Chancellor frequently circumvented the budget review process. Often last to find out there were new bills to be paid, the VC-RMP's office worked largely in reaction mode until the early 1990s. As before, the Medical Center and the Schools continued their own separate resource planning.

In the same period, UCSF grew mightily, by all quantitative measures—research dollars, clinical dollars, patient population, faculty, staff, etc. Its complexity grew also, as it managed large campuses and populations at San Francisco General, the VA and Mt Zion Medical Centers, and the Laurel Heights and Mission Center campuses, plus research operations—basic, clinical, wetlab, dry-lab—at multiple sites.

In sharp contrast, UCSF's executive management structure hardly differed from that of the 1950s. Consultations took place in a virtual black box: faced with a possible decision, the Chancellor requested advice from a few individuals, who might include a prime stakeholder. This private meeting would then produce a decision, often issued with little explanation and scanty records of details or rationale. Sometimes staff were asked to analyze problems, but formal presentations were few. No comprehensive financial planning took place, but the Chancellor or his Senior Vice Chancellor made financial decisions and funds were allocated. This process may have reflected decades of rising NIH budgets and a generous legislature, making budget plans and careful analysis of long-term decisions appear superfluous. Just as likely, a management structure entrenched in the past preferred not to notice stark harbingers of change.

A Perfect Storm

In FY1991, the state of California was afflicted by a major recession, regarded at the time as the largest since the Great Depression. Between FY1991 and FY1995, the state reduced UCSF's funding by $38M, or ~26% in comparison to FY1991 (12). Suddenly, the Schools and the Chancellor's office(s) faced a scary reduction in their major funding source. The state largely funded faculty and staffs of the Schools of Dentistry, Nursing, and Pharmacy, which otherwise had only small sources of clinical and other income. The School of Medicine, with substantial clinical and sponsored income, still had to absorb this 26% reduction in state funds, and managed to do so at the time from other resources. But this manageable crisis served as a frightening harbinger of a perfect storm that would sharply disrupt habits, customs, and practices inherited from prosperous earlier times and produce challenges that still persist today.

The recession's economic effects coincided with a quite separate storm in 1991, which originated at Stanford, when an on-site federal auditor alleged that Stanford was defrauding the federal government in recovering ICR for its research. While the actual sin turned out to be little more than sloppy cost accounting, a public brouhaha (see chapter 3) led the federal government to change a basic rule of OMB Circular A-21, sharply reducing universities' ability to charge certain support costs (e.g., telephones, some staff) directly to research grants. At the time when the new A-21 rules took effect, internal estimates indicated that UCSF Schools would need to find about $12 million annually to replace the support previously paid from direct costs (12).

In addition, in these years President Clinton was fighting budget wars with Congress. The resulting continuing resolutions meant that already allocated grants and contracts were reduced to 90% of the dollars initially approved, and new grant funds were held in abeyance (sometimes for months) until each annual budget battle was resolved. To make the future look even less certain, the health care marketplace was also in an uproar, agitated in part by the Clinton administration's attempt to implement a modified form of single-payer health care, but even more by the health care industry's forays into managed care. Suddenly, tertiary and quaternary care centers like UCSF appeared to have been transformed from institutional cash cows into cost centers. At one point in the 1990s, an executive of a large Health Maintenance Organization (HMO) told an audience of UCSF department chairs that UCSF's clinical enterprise would rapidly shrink within the coming decade, as more competitive and efficient HMOs would capture its patients (13).

In today's world, UCSF knows how to weather such crises and threats, but in the mid-1990s managers of the UCSF Campus were not prepared to deal with a continuing state budget crisis, and new federal regulations, which combined to produce a revenue loss of nearly $50M per year in 1995. Never exposed to such troubles, administrators had no process in place to deal with budget cuts, big or small. Now they began to recognize that UCSF must learn how to assess its resources, plan their future use, and make critical decisions— and must, in each case, include the entire UCSF enterprise. Separate, nearly independent financial silos—hospitals, schools, and the chancellor's office— would have to learn how to work together.

Centralized Resource Planning: the Maiden Voyage

A new Chancellor, Joseph Martin, took the helm at UCSF in 1993, following a career at Harvard Medical School and four years (1989-93) as Dean of UCSF's School of Medicine. As Chancellor, this "new broom" quickly ordered formation of a financial plan for the CCF (Campus Core Funds) and a process for making decisions about resources that cut across all the institution's silos. In 1994 the Chancellor's Office produced the first Chancellor's Financial Plan (CFP) and announced formation of an Executive Budget Committee (EBC). Today these are called the Core Financial Plan (CFP) and the Budget & Investment (B&I) Committee.

In 1994 the CFP comprised the first comprehensive examination of all resources directly managed by the Chancellor's Office, plus a planning forecast for future years, complete with assumptions and analysis. Because the CFP did not yet include revenues and expenses of the Medical Center or the four Schools, the old decentralized model remained intact, although the Chancellor had always been charged with overall responsibility for all UCSF's resources. The EBC's composition constituted the first real step to change the decentralized model: its co-chairs were leaders in positions now termed Executive Vice Chancellor-Provost (EVCP) and Senior Vice Chancellor-Finance & Administration (SVCFA); its initial members were the CEO of the Medical

Center and deans of the four Schools; later its members also included the dean of the Graduate Division and the chair of the Academic Senate. Staffed by the Chancellor's Budget and Resource Management office, the EBC had four main functions:

1. To serve as a sounding board for institution-wide resource planning issues.
2. To coordinate intra-campus resource issues.
3. To conduct annual reviews of the resources and initiatives of each major budget "Control Point"—including the four Schools, the Medical Center, and the Chancellor's office and its two major units (offices of the EVCP and the SVCFA).
4. To provide advice on setting priorities for the Chancellor's central resources.

The CFP gradually became a successful new model for UCSF, because the Chancellor put on the table central resources for both enterprise-wide initiatives and needs of individual Control Points. The new annual budget review process required each Control Point to present its budget, discuss resource problems and issues, new revenue strategies, and new programmatic directions—that is, challenges they had to confront, future goals, and how they planned to manage them. To help set funding priorities, their needs for resources were on the table and evaluated in comparison with other needs. The perfect storm's crises showed Control Point leaders both the limits of each other's resources and the need for enterprise-wide planning. For the first time, a uniform formula reallocated some ICR dollars to help Schools respond to the new A-21 rules, and Schools reeling from state budget cuts had a place to present their needs and receive support funds. The EBC provided key stakeholders a forum to discuss institution-wide issues and balancing capital needs vs. operating requirements. Importantly, all resource decisions were also documented in formal allocation letters, which contained the allocation's rationale and specified spending rules, reporting requirements, or milestones. From then on, every Chancellor's funding decisions were documented in this way.

Paradoxically, the Medical Center's ill-fated merger with Stanford's Medical Center—beginning in 1996 and unwound in 2000—improved the new cooperative enterprise-wide model: when the Medical Center returned to the UCSF fold, its previous management was replaced by a new team, headed by CEO Mark Laret; freed from past baggage, it could build new ways of business planning.

UCSF's new tools for managing resources and planning (the CFP) and an enterprise-wide consultative body (the EBC) would serve the campus well through good and bad times to come. Thus, just as the Campus was implementing programs and finances for research at Mission Bay campus (2001-04), yet another financial crisis (the "dot-com bust") led to further cuts in state funding. For UCSF, the unkindest cut was the state's decision not to provide ~$14M per year to maintain buildings and supply utilities for its newly emerging research campus (*14*). This loss did slow the project, but fortunately campus leaders and the EBC had advance notice, plus tools for making decisions based on data rather than guesses to adjust CFP dollars and realign necessary resources.

The Ten-Year Forecast Model

UCSF's first enterprise-wide forecast (in 2012) can be traced to collapse of a hospital in a 1994 California earthquake, long before that forecast appeared. By the 21st century, resulting changes in state seismic laws (SB 1953) for hospitals meant that UCSF's Mt. Zion and Moffitt Hospitals, would either have to be re-built from the inside out or replaced. Because it would cost less to build another hospital (and find another conforming use for the Mt. Zion and Moffitt buildings), and such a hospital could not be built at Parnassus, attention focused on Mission Bay. Realizing that separate silo-based models would not suffice to gain UC Regents' approval, in 2006 planners for the Chancellor and the Medical Center engaged an outside firm to help build a joint UCSF financial model for preparing consolidated 10-year financial forecasts (*15*).

By 2009 the model was built and tested, but two additional years were required to fully integrate the medical center and the Campus and include specific financial plans and assumptions from the four Schools—that is, to refine each entity's plans to fit into the model and develop shared methods, charts of accounts and classification categories, so as to forge a seamless fit between the financial reports of each and the overall forecast model. The first forecast was published in draft in 2011. After further refinements, the comprehensive UCSF financial plan and 10-year forecast was first published in 2012—and again every year since, improving in clarity and precision with each iteration.

While this comprehensive financial planning and modeling tool was under development, another financial crisis struck: the financial crash of 2008-9 and the subsequent recession again reduced state funds for education, as the Governor cut almost $1B (more than 25%) from UC's budget. For UCSF, this crisis reduced resources to their very limits, owing to cumulative effect of many years of state funding reductions, plus development and operation of a new major campus at Mission Bay. Fortunately, however, by this time the EBC had dealt with resource problems for 15 years, and Control Points had learned how to work jointly in making hard decisions. Staff sought redundancies and organizational combinations as potential opportunities to reduce costs. Control Point plans were shared, so a cut in one place didn't produce unanticipated consequences elsewhere. Ultimately, one offshoot of the EBC process, a painful exercise euphemistically dubbed Operational Excellence (OE), eliminated more than 400 Campus employees (16). The goal of this exercise was not simply to reduce costs, but—more specifically—to respond to substantial decreases in state support. Overall, OE did achieve ~$50M in annual savings (run-rate savings, rather than one time savings; 16) and UCSF weathered the financial storm. Inevitably, of course, some departments experienced losses in quality of staff services, while others enjoyed gains. Human resource activities and processing of contracts and grants were re-shaped into new models, with results that differed in different departments, based on their previous handling of both these functions: thus, in some cases costs charged to departments for both functions actually increased; others received better services than they had before OE was instituted. The OE process tried hard to mitigate deleterious effects of workload shifts, with success in some cases but not in others. Unfortunately, however, some departments experienced a loss of services or found themselves paying more than before, and deemed OE a futile and damaging exercise. Impacts of the cuts in state support and the OE response to those cuts are still being felt, as we shall see in later discussions of inadequate support for faculty salaries and research administration (chapters 7-9, below).

Current Decision-making and the 2015 Financial Plan and Forecast

Luckily, UCSF's development has been guided by a strong mix of entrepreneurs, visionary thinkers, and good stewards, who consistently found ways to move in the right directions as conditions changed, for more than half a century. In a further stroke of good fortune, a combination of new financial resources and economic threats fostered gradual development of effective processes for analysis, planning, and making long-term decisions. Shaped by a 20-year baptism of fire, the process is still changing.

That said, it is fair to ask pointed questions. Where, exactly, do decisions regarding high level, longer-term issues take place? In actual practice, who thinks hard about such issues and makes decisions that, for instance:

1. Choose among alternative paths for future directions of research at UCSF?
2. Commit UCSF to expanding one major activity or contracting another?
3. Take account of possible impacts of politics on government funding, and hedge bets with respect to academic missions—research and teaching—as well as patient care?
4. Determine whether and when to issue hundreds of millions of dollars in debt, to be repaid over 30-40 years, backed by a source of funding (ICR) that is exquisitely sensitive to political influence?
5. Mitigate (or, ignore) the burden of soft-money salaries for UCSF research faculty.
6. Seek to improve the quality of training for basic scientists and clinician-scientists (rather than simply continuing to pay the growing costs of training)?

From the first part of this chapter, one might surmise that such decisions are made by the Chancellor, in combination with the EBC—now called the B&I Committee—and by deans of the Schools, in collaboration with their parallel planning experts. After all, the scope of the B&I Committee and its offshoot, an informal working group of financial officers called the B&I Working Group is to manage buttons and switches that control the flow of resources, including decisions that judge trade-offs among strategic invest-ments, allocations for ongoing activities, and large-scale outlays for capital, information technology, and programs (*17*). Both the B&I Committee and its Working Group are designed to bring transparency to the budgeting process and allow Control Point leaders to have their say in setting priorities and man-aging critical trade-offs.

The truth, as always, is more complex. In reality, senior leaders largely decide which decisions will be examined, analyzed, and implemented by the B&I committee. In order to do so, they must be able to communicate freely their hopes and fears with respect to any new idea, long-term decision, or major policy change before it becomes public knowledge. But because UCSF is—in reality if not in funding—a public institution, there Is a critical tension between the institution's duty and need to be trusted by the public, on the one hand, and freedom of communication among leaders, on the other. To manage that tension, UCSF's Chancellor meets regularly for critical discus-sions with an Executive Cabinet, composed of a more limited set of senior leaders—the Chancellor, the UCSF Health CEO, deans of the four Schools, the EVCP, the SVCFA and the UCSF Counsel. Minutes are not kept and no agendas are prepared. Sometimes these discussions require the presence of attorneys, so the attorney-client privilege can allow free communication among leaders. Once a decision is agreed upon and action becomes necessary, UCSF makes its further discussion and implementation public, at the right time and at the right level—often first at the B&I/Working Group level, and then to the Campus and the public. Decisions are thus ultimately more open than at private universities, but UCSF's gradual disclosure process shares with those universities one hitch, which is probably irremediable: only decisions that are slated for implementation are revealed; so, if high-level leaders decide not to make a decision, no one else may ever know. Clearly, however, failure to make decisions can produce disasters—in war, governments, large institutions, and even our daily lives.

UCSF's financial outcome in FY2014 was good (see chapters 1-3), but the outcome in FY2015 was even better—and better than most people suspected, as indicated in the most recent 10-year UCSF financial plan and forecast, in 2015 (1), and in the annual financial report summary previewed in October, 2015 (18). Between the 2014 and 2015 forecasts, the new Mission Bay hospitals became operational, clarifying previous uncertainties. Other key comparisons reflect positive changes:

1. Investment strategies (e.g., the TRIP program and other cash management changes, begun in 2008 and bearing real fruit since 2010) had a banner year in 2015, earning ~$60 million more than in 2014, based largely on a $51 million capital accumulation payout (18).
2. The medical faculty earned income on professional services agreements (PSA) was $32 million higher than 2014 (18).
3. UCSF Health had substantially higher revenue—a net increase of $105 million more than the previous forecast—and higher operating expenses than expected (18). This resulted in a small $14M increase in the Strategic Support UCSF Health could transfer to the Campus (18).
4. Unrestricted cash reserves continued to grow and are projected to increase by more than 50% at the end of the 10 year forecast period (1).

Nonetheless, potentially daunting issues must be considered. One is the projected growth of debt largely backed by ICR, which will increase from slightly more than $1B at the end of FY2014 to more than $1.8B by 2020. Consequently, annual payments from ICR will grow to more than $140M per year and remain near that level until FY2035. If UCSF continues to earn ~$200M per year in total ICR, about 70% of that ICR will be consumed each year to pay off debts.

UCSF's remarkable ability to attract awards for sponsored research (and associated ICR; see chapter 3) persisted over the past decade, despite a substantial overall tightening of federal funds for research. While UCSF's research grew, that of many other academic research institutions declined. If the federal government's largesse fails to increase or even declines (either is more likely than sustained long-term support; *19*), will UCSF's research growth continue in the face of declining research funds at other institutions? To commit 70% of potentially tenuous ICR to 30-plus years of debt payments appears a bold act of faith.

Moreover, UCSF has devised no concrete, mid-to-long-term strategy for dealing with unexpected surges in revenue, like that of 2015, which is expected to repeat in 2016. The recent 10-year plan and forecast (*1*) pay lip service to developing new revenue for the campus and reducing operating costs, but, on the surface, they essentially toss the recent unanticipated increase in revenues back into the central money pool. (A high-ranking UCSF official informed us that some of this surplus was indeed moved into a general endowment-like fund.) Instead, we suggest that UCSF adopt a clear, well-publicized, long-term strategy for investing "extra" revenues into a General Endowment that can be used to deal with future cuts in state funding support or to backstop ICR funds currently used for debt payments.

Before closing this chapter, consider this question: as it invests in the programs, buildings, and people necessary for its future, how can an academic research institution like UCSF avoid the kind of financial over-reach that could place it at the edge of a financial cliff without a rescue net? Institutional leaders aver that part of their job is to keep such risks under firm control.

Nonetheless, institutional leaders frequently are subjected to intense pressures from a rich donor to build a facility or house a program that is not a top priority of the institution and will unavoidably incur additional hidden costs the donor will not pay. Let us consider a hypothetical example of a $300M building, to be named for a rich donor who pays one third of the building cost. Here are some of the hidden costs the institution will have to pay:

1. *The remaining construction cost* will be paid by the university, which must find additional donors, commit significant amounts of its own reserves, or issue new debt (for which it will pay ~$12M a year to service a $200M loan).

2. The annual *costs of operating and maintaining the building* (including utilities,

custodial service, security, equipment maintenance, maintaining information technology systems, etc.). Such costs can amount annually to $25-30 per gross square foot (gsf)—or, for a 250,000 gsf building, $6.2-7.5M every year.

3. The institution will have to recruit new faculty to fulfill the program envisioned by the donor. *Initial recruitment costs* alone for faculty investigators of real quality may come to $2-5M per person; a building that requires 30 new investigators will incur start-up costs amounting to $100-200M.

For such a building, the university will pay hidden costs, amounting over the building's first decade to ~$340M (including $120M for debt service, $70M for building maintenance, and $150M for recruiting faculty). Thus, if the donor's gift is to produce real benefits, the institution will pay a yearly average extra cost of $34M a year over the first 10 years after the building opens. This conservative estimate does not include additional costs, such as salary and benefits for investigators and costs of hiring and paying administrative staff. Moreover, as described in chapter 4, indirect costs on research grants awarded to investigators in the building will not fully compensate for these costs during its first decade.

Finally, the decision to pay for such a building will mean that UCSF incurs significant opportunity costs: lacking the $340M it has chose to pay for the donor's building, UCSF must defer or not fund other programs or buildings. Because such lost opportunities can prove significant for determining UCSF's future, leaders must ensure that each major investment in a building or program is the right thing to do. The process of making decisions about distribution of scarce resources is only as good as the rigor imposed by those charged with the responsibility for it. The 10-year resource plan that UCSF engages in each year is a detailed and thoughtful process, currently with solid financial planners and analysts and executive decision makers riding herd on it. Both authors of this book have seen outside pressure from donors that produces real mischief, but in the long run the institution has usually built a first class facility that works for 75 years or more. Every year UCSF's leaders face similarly daunting gambles. As for the payoff, in each case, only time will really tell.

Subsequent chapters explore the funding future of research in greater detail, particularly with respect to paying research faculty salaries. Chapter 10 will revisit several questions raised in the present chapter. The underlying issues are critical for UCSF and all health science research institutions.

Chapter 6

Researchers' salaries: Soft dollars, thorny issues

At UCSF and other large institutions, salaries inevitably become the hot-button issue for everyone, from top leaders to the lowest-paid workers. Salaries are usually by far the institution's biggest expense: UCSF's $2.773B in expenditures for salary and benefits together account for 65% of total annual expenditures ($4.290B in FY2014; Table 6-1; chapter 1; *1*). More viscerally, each employee wants very much to know how much he/she will earn every year, what benefits are covered, for how long the salary will last, whether and how it may increase, and where it comes from—and asks the same questions about colleagues. The answers strongly influence employees' satisfaction with their work and the institution, their attitudes toward the institution's missions, and their interactions with and loyalty toward co-workers, leaders, students, and patients.

This chapter concentrates on salaries of UCSF's employees. Employee headcounts and salary dollars reflect the institution's strengths, but also raise thorny issues. One of the thorniest derives from the large proportion of faculty salaries paid from research grants, rather than by UCSF or the clinical enterprise. Such "soft-money" salaries keep research afloat, but pose difficult conundrums for UCSF's future.

Big picture

To understand more complex issues, we first consider salaries of different sets of UCSF employees and sketch the numerous and diverse subsets of UCSF's faculty.

Headcounts and dollars. In FY2014 UCSF paid $2.138B in salary to a workforce of nearly 23,000 people (Table 6-1); Campus or clinical enterprise employees make up, respectively, 63% or 37% of the total workforce and receive similar percentages of salary payments. Of all UCSF employees, more than half (52%) are staff represented by unions—including nurses, other patient

Table 6-1. Salary and benefits at UCSF (FY2014)*

	Staff			Fac-ulty	Acad. Non-fac.	Totals
	Rep.	Non-rep.	Temp.			
Campus						
Headcount	5,621	4,414		2,545	2,391	14,971
Total salary ($M)	285	352		532	138	1,307
Mean salary ($ thou)	51	80		209	58	
Total benefits ($M)						348
Benefits, % of salary						27
Clinical enterprise						
Headcount	6,280	1,677				7,957
Total salary ($M)	596	192	31			819
Mean salary ($ thou)	95	114				
Total benefits ($M)						261
Benefits, % of salary						32
UCSF (consolidated)						
Headcount	11,901	6,091		2,545	2,391	22,928
Total salary ($M)	881	544	31	532	138	2,138
Total benefits ($M)						635
Total salary + benefits ($M)						2,773

*Headcounts are as of June 30, 2014; benefits include UC retirement plan, retiree health benefits, health insurance, social security/medicare, worker's compensation, and other. Union-represented (Rep.) staff include those engaged in health care, research support, administration, lab work as postdocs, patient care & service, nursing, non-senate academic research. Unrepresented staff (Non-rep.) include individuals in senior management, management services, professional support, and non-faculty academic employees (academic coordinators, lecturers, post-doctoral scholars, residents and graduate students). Data is from reference 1.

care workers, laboratory research personnel, postdoctoral scholars, and others; together this group received about 41% of UCSF's total salary bill, at mean annual wages of $51,000 (Campus) and $95,000 (clinical enterprise). Staff not represented by unions account for 27% of UCSF employees and receive 26% of total salary; this group includes senior managers and professional and support staff, earning mean yearly salaries of $80,000 (Campus) or $114,000 (clinical enterprise). Academic non-faculty employees (including academic co-ordinators, lecturers, hospital resident physicians, postdoctoral scholars, and graduate students) comprise 10% of the UCSF workforce and earn 6.1% of total salary paid, for a mean annual wage of $58,000. Finally, UCSF's academic faculty (11% of workforce, 25% of total salary) earns a mean annual wage of $209,000.

In addition to $2.138B in salaries, UCSF also paid $635M (29.7% of salary, on average, across all UCSF) in benefits, including the UC retirement plan, health benefits, Social Security, Medicare, and worker's compensation. As discussed in chapter 2, benefit costs increased considerably over the past

Table 6-2. Faculty series: numbers, expectations and privileges*‡

	Ladder Rank	In Residence	Clinical X	Adjunct	Health Sci Clinical
Number of individuals	333	458	422	398	784
Total UCSF salary ($M)+	87	102	120	44	139
Avg.+ yearly salary ($thou)+	261	223	285	111	177
Expectations					
Research	+++	+++	++	+++ + or + +++	+
Teaching	+++	+++	+++	+ +++	+++
Prof.+	+++	+++	+++	+	+++
competence Service	+++	+++	+	+	+
Privileges					
Acad.+ senate membership	Yes	Yes	Yes	No***	No***
% Time	100	100	100	Any	Any
Sabbatical leave	Yes	P.L.P+	P.L.P+	Rare¶	Rare¶
Duration of appointment§	Tenure	Yearly/ Unlimited**	Yearly	Yearly	Yearly

*For a summary of expectations and privileges that apply to the clinical series at UCSF, see reference 3. Sources of data on numbers and UCSF salaries of individuals in these series (FY2014) are described in reference 4.

¶Professional leave may sometimes be allowed as an exception

§For faculty without tenure, all appointments must be renewed yearly, except that in residence associate or full Professor appointments have no end date.

‡Abbreviations: Acad., Academic; Avg., average; Health Sci, Health Sciences; $M, millions of dollars; P.L.P. = "professional leave possible"; Prof., professional; $thou, thousands of dollars

five years, mainly owing to a gap between projected funding of the retirement system and actuarial assessment of future retirement obligation liability. Consequently, UC decided to tax campuses for the funds needed to maintain pension support (*2*).

What exactly is a faculty member? UCSF faculty members belong to several many-splendored species. Faced with multiple and ever-changing needs for faculty with widely diverse expertise and goals, the ever-fertile academic imagination has invented no fewer than five distinct "series" of faculty for UCSF. [As a bonus, the University defines a kind of shadow series, "Academic non-faculty," that comprises 2,391 employees (Table 6-1) who are not faculty at all!] The rationale for the five bona fide faculty series is to define two kinds of relations between the institution and its faculty (*3*). First, for each series, the university describes the relative importance of four categories of qualifications and contributions it considers in judging whether individual faculty in the series should advance in academic rank (Table 6-2). These categories include research, teaching, professional activity and competence (as a research scientist and/or, if the faculty member is a health-care provider, as clinicians), and University and public service (termed "service" in Table 6-2). Second, relations between faculty and the University are described in terms of the privileges and rules individuals in each faculty series may expect the university to apply to them. Some of these rules and privileges (Table 6-2) include: membership (or not) in the UCSF Academic Senate, a representative body whose members advise the administration and vote on academic issues; whether the appointment must be full-time (100%) or may be part-time; whether series members can take sabbatical leave; and duration of a faculty member's appointment, which can range, depending on faculty series, from one year to "tenure," as described below.

Ladder-rank faculty. This is one of three faculty series that contribute most substantially to UCSF's research mission. UCSF's 333 ladder-rank faculty members make up 13% of all its faculty (Table 6-2; *4*). They advance in academic rank based on equally weighted judgments of research accomplishments and teaching prowess, and typically direct independent research in laboratories, clinical settings, or both; their research is usually funded by grant support from federal and/or private sources. They are also called "tenure-track" faculty because the University contributes to their salary from its own coffers (and thus not only from research grants, clinical income, or contracts with external agencies) and because promotion to associate professor rank raises them to tenure (Table 6-2).

As a term, "tenure" means different things at different institutions, and its meanings have changed dramatically over time, at UCSF and elsewhere. The tenured security of ladder-rank UCSF faculty in the 1970s, 80s, and early 90s depended critically on the University's then correct assurance that it would pay a substantial fraction of their salaries. This assurance began when they were accorded ladder-rank status as assistant professors, continued thereafter if they were awarded tenure, and terminated only with the faculty member's voluntary retirement or resignation, involuntary dismissal, or death. In the 1970s, tenure-track faculty members of basic science departments received ~75% of their salary—called a "Full-Time Equivalent," or FTE—from the University, which they supplemented by an additional ~25% paid from research grants. In clinical departments, ladder-rank faculty members received the same FTE dollars as did basic science faculty members at the same rank, but usually maintained higher total salaries with supplements from both grants and clinical income. In those days UCSF received state educational appropriations large enough to pay FTE salary and benefits of every ladder-rank faculty member, plus those of many administrative staff. Today, UCSF's average ladder-rank faculty researcher receives only 27% of her/his salary from state instructional funds, as a later table in this chapter will show.

By the mid-1990s this cozy arrangement had begun to deteriorate: State support for faculty and administrative salaries decreased—slowly at first, then faster—as the economy faltered in the early 1990s and taxpayers complained about paying for education. As FTE dollars for ladder-rank faculty became scarcer, they were replaced by money from multiple sources: higher supplements from (i) research grants (in basic science departments, almost always) and/or (ii) clinical income (in clinical departments), plus (iii) whatever funds department chairs, deans and chancellors could squeeze from endowments and budgets. Diminished FTE support and UCSF's responses to it profoundly altered the institution.

The erosion of tenure at UCSF parallels situations in most US medical schools, owing largely to big increases in numbers of clinical faculty and reduction in dollars available to pay them. Nationally, the relative reduction in tenured faculty has been especially severe for MD faculty in clinical departments of those schools (5): in such departments, since 1984, the number of tenured MD faculty has remained at or below ~20,000 since 1984, while the number of untenured faculty increased about six-fold (from ~8,000 to ~56,000); the proportion of tenured faculty consequently fell from 60% to less than 25%. Moreover, the financial security associated with tenure deteriorated over the same time period (6).

In residence faculty. Numbering 458, or 18% of all UCSF faculty (4), individuals in this series advance in rank depending on criteria weighted just like those of ladder-rank faculty (Table 6-2). In residence faculty are not promised support from the institution, but instead "must generate the funding for their salary from contracts and grants, and/or clinical activities, or receive a salary from an affiliated institution" (7). In this series promotions to associate professor carry no whiff of tenure: appointments of assistant professors in residence must be renewed every year; appointments at higher ranks have no end date, but if funds to support a faculty member's salary are not available, a department may formally impose a "term appointment, . . . [with] a minimum of twelve months of support at the level of retirement-covered compensation" (7). Thus in residence faculty members are very much on their own, and usually pay 90% or more of their salary from a combination of research grants and clinical income. In consequence, most in residence faculty are located in clinical departments.

Adjunct faculty. Faculty in this series, numbering 398 (16% of all faculty; 4), earn advancement in rank by criteria weighted differently from those applied to the two series discussed above. Specifically, adjunct faculty can be promoted primarily for their contributions in either teaching, with minimal research, or in research, with minimal teaching. As teachers, they may run courses in basic science departments; as researchers, most PhD adjunct faculty are located in clinical departments, less often in basic science departments. Often, but not always, adjunct researchers work under the direction of other faculty and do not conduct fully independent research programs. They usually receive lower salaries (at any rank) than ladder-rank or in residence faculty, are appointed for one year at a time, can work part-time, and lack privileges like Academic Senate membership and sabbatical leave.

Two series limited to clinical faculty. These series contribute relatively less than the others less to UCSF's research mission. Primary responsibilities of the 422 faculty members (17% of all faculty; *3, 7*) in the professor of Clinical X series (where "X" stands for the specialty of a clinical department—e.g., radiology, urology, ophthalmology, etc.) are teaching and clinical work, but they also engage in "creative activities," including research. Health sciences clinical professors (784 faculty, or 31% of all UCSF faculty) make up the largest of all the five faculty series. They include hospitalists and other clinicians in UCSF's clinical enterprise who qualify for advancement primarily on the basis of teaching and clinical work, but may also engage in research and university and public service; like adjunct faculty, members of this latter series may work less than 100% time. Faculty in both these series are appointed on a yearly basis. For details, see Table 6-2 and reference *2*.

Finances, culture, and expansion. Faculty in basic science and clinical departments (*8*) responded very differently to losing state support for faculty salaries, although the losses afflicted both at the same time. Most UCSF faculty in basic science departments are in the ladder-rank series, and over many decades became accustomed to substantial salary support from state dollars. As PhDs, most are not able to supplement their salaries with clinical income. Consequently, most basic science departments did not increase numbers of their research faculty beyond the number of FTEs previously paid from generous state support; now they find it increasingly difficult to garner support for recruiting new faculty, even for positions vacated by retirement. In contrast, clinical departments continued in the same years to expand their research activities, recruiting new faculty researcher-clinicians at both junior and senior levels. Between 2004 and 2014, UCSF's clinical departments increased their research support—federal, private, and total combined—by 73%, while support for basic science departments and Organized Research Units (ORUs) from the same sources increased only 11-18%, as chapter 7 will show in greater detail (*9*).

Differing sources available to pay researcher salaries led basic science and clinical researchers to develop different academic cultures. For decades, the former (mostly PhDs) received modestly lower average salaries, for which they depended primarily on state educational funds; now many of them consider having to pay more of their salary from grants an unwarranted time- and energy-consuming distraction from serious research. In the same decades, numbers of MD faculty in clinical departments increased as the clinical enterprise expanded. Consequently, the gradual decline in university dollars for salary support has reduced the proportion of clinical faculty (i.e., ladder rank faculty) who receive any salary from the institution, and the university contributes smaller fractions of salary to those who do. Many who play large roles in clinical teaching must seek most of their salary from clinical revenues, and those who play large roles in research (especially ladder rank and in residence faculty) predominantly support their salaries from research grants and from clinical revenues. Adjunct faculty in clinical departments (many of whom are PhDs) previously obtained large fractions of their salary from grants, and continue to do so.

The effects of different cultures were potentiated by other influences that favored expansion of clinical departments and clinical research. Of these the most critical was the abundant and persistent financial success of the health care industry, which has expanded faster than most of the US economy (see chapter 1). In keeping with that success, NIH funding has tilted away from basic investigation of biological mechanisms and toward large grants oriented toward goals considered more clinically relevant. In addition, increased private research funding for the most part supports research aimed at diagnosis and treatment of human disease. The tilt toward the clinic strongly influences academic researchers, leaders, and philanthropic donors at UCSF and elsewhere (see chapters 7-10).

Salary sources for research faculty

Of UCSF's faculty in FY2014 (i.e., defined as faculty by belonging to a specific faculty series; *4*)—1,498 received at least some portion of their salaries from a research grant or contract with a federal or a private source, philanthropic or industrial (Table 6-3; *10*). Thus of UCSF's 2,545 faculty members (Table 6-1), 59% were "sponsored" faculty—i.e., engaged in research and paid, at least in part, by a sponsoring source. All salary for the "unsponsored" 41% came from clinical income and/or other UCSF coffers. Overall, sponsored faculty re-

Table 6-3. Faculty who receive sponsored salary support: Departments, rank, age, and series*

Category	Headcount		Salary (all sources)		Sponsored salary		
	No.	%	Total ($M)	Avg yearly ($thou)	Total ($M)	Avg yearly ($thou)	% of all salary[¶]
All spons[§] faculty	1498	100	302	202	114	68	38
Dept type							
Clinical	1223	82	254	208	89	73	35
Basic science	197	13	34	173	17	88	51
ORU	73	5	13	177	7.6	104	59
Other	5	0.3	0.98	196	0.18	36	19
Rank							
Instr *or* Asst	463	31	65	140	29	62	44
Associate	358	24	66	184	26	73	39
Professor	677	45	171	253	59	88	35
Age <40	318	21	49	155	19	59	38
40>Age<50	545	36	103	189	42	76	41
Age >50	635	42	150	236	54	84	36
Series							
Ladder-rank	282	19	75	267	24	86	32
In Residence	408	27	90	221	40	98	45
Clinical X	211	14	4	258	11	52	20
Adjunct	349	23	40	114	28	81	71
Health Sci Clin	249	17	43	172	10	41	24

*Data in this table (*10*) pertain to the 1,498 UCSF faculty members who were (i) explicitly designated as belonging to a particular faculty series (*4*) and also (ii) obtained at least some part of their salaries from sponsored projects. Twelve departments are classified as basic science departments, and 26 as clinical departments (*8*).

¶% of all salary in the category on the left (e.g., in the second row of data: 35% of total salary of sponsored faculty in clinical departments, or, in the last row of data: 24% of total salary of all sponsored faculty in the HS Clinical series).

§Abbreviations: spons, sponsored; $M, millions of dollars; $ thou, thousands of dollars; ORU, Organized Research Units, such as the Cardiovascular Research Institute, the Cancer Research Institute, and others; Instr, instructor; Asst, assistant professor; Clinical X, Professor of Clinical X series (where X is a clinical department); Health Sci Clinical, Health Science Clinical Professor series.

ceived $114M from sponsoring sources—that is, 38% of all UCSF salary they received, and 21% of the $532M in total salary UCSF paid its faculty (sponsored and unsponsored; see Tables 6-1 and 6-3) in FY2014. Sponsored faculty received a total of $148M from sponsored sources, if we include $114M in take-home salary plus ~29.7%, or ~$34M, in benefits.

Now we are ready to examine the gross distributions of sponsored salary among faculty ranks, age, and series, as well as departments (Table 6-3), and compare the relative amounts of salary faculty received from sponsoring and other sources (Table 6-4). Then we shall consider distributions of salary sources among deciles of sponsored faculty who receive different percentages of their salary from sponsoring sources (Figures 6-1 to 6-3).

Gross distributions of sponsored salary. Among academic departments, the distributions of sponsored and unsponsored faculty are not surprising. While virtually every faculty member in a basic science department or an Organized Research Unit (ORU) is sponsored, both types of unit are small; consequently, their faculty account for only 13% or 5%, respectively, of all sponsored faculty, while the remaining 82% of sponsored faculty are in clinical departments (Table 6-3). Clinical departments also contain a large proportion of unsponsored faculty (41% of their total of 2,076 faculty; *10*).

Sponsored faculty members are distributed asymmetrically among faculty series at UCSF, in keeping with the defined role (Table 6-3) of each series. Based on headcounts of total faculty (Table 6-2) and sponsored faculty (Table 6-3), the proportions of faculty members who receive some portion of salary from sponsored sources were 89% for in residence, 88% for adjunct, 85% for ladder-rank, 50% for Clinical X, and 32% for Health Science Clinical. These data correlate with the relative importance of research prowess for advancement in the in residence and ladder-rank series. Within the adjunct series, the data indicate that researchers outnumber teachers (promotion in this series may depend predominantly on either research prowess or teaching). Sponsored salary goes to smaller proportions of faculty In the clinical X (50%) and health science clinical series (32%), which place less relative emphasis on research as an absolute criterion for promotion. If we focus instead on subsets of faculty who receive sponsored salary in each series, we see parallel results. Thus the sponsored faculty in the two predominantly clinical series, Professor of Clinical X and Research Sciences Clinical, receive relatively low percentages of total salary from sponsored sources (20% and 24%, respectively), as compared to sponsored in residence or ladder-rank faculty (45% and 32%, respectively). Sponsored adjunct faculty receive by far the highest percentage of salary (71%) from sponsored sources.

Other data in Table 6-3 (focusing only on faculty with some sponsored salary) also confirm inferences any knowledgeable observer of UCSF's faculty might make: (i) faculty in clinical departments are not only more numerous than those in basic science departments or ORUs, they also (on average) receive modestly higher average individual salaries and garner lower percentages of salary from sponsored sources; (ii) on average, faculty who are older or at higher academic ranks receive more salary; (iii) average yearly salaries are highest for ladder-rank ($267,000) and clinical X faculty ($258,000), lowest for adjunct faculty ($114,000), and intermediate for in residence ($221,000) and health science clinical faculty ($172,000).

Most sponsored faculty members receive salary from other sources as

Table 6-4. Sponsored salary, overall by source*[§]

Salary source	Spons	Instr	Clin	G/E	Other
Headcount (with some $ from source)	1498	564	1064	577	367
% with some $ from source	100	38	71	39	25
Total salary $ paid (all sources, $M)	302	130	246	123	78
Avg individual yearly salary (all sources, $thou)	201	230	231	214	212
Total *sponsored* salary ($M)	114	44	77	49	29
Mean annual *sponsored* salary for faculty who also earn salary from the source in this column ($thou)	76	78	73	85	80
Mean % *sponsored* salary for people who also get salary from source in this column	38	34	32	38	38
Total salary $ from this column's source for headcount in this column ($M)	114	35	124	22	7.9
Mean annual salary from source in this column ($thou)	76	61	117	38	21
Mean % salary from source in column	38	27	51	18	10

*In FY2014, all faculty in this Table belonged to a defined faculty series (4) and received at least part of their salary from a sponsoring source (10). Note that in each horizontal row the headcounts and percentages do not add up to 100%; this is because virtually every faculty member who received money from sponsored sources also received dollars from one or two or even three additional sources.

§Abbreviations: Spons = sponsored; Instr = instructional; Clin (aka S&S); G/E = gifts & endowments.

well (Table 6-4). The population of all 1,498 sponsored faculty in FY2014 garnered an average $76,000 per year from sponsored sources (38% of their mean yearly salary; Tables 6-3 and 6-4). Individual sponsored faculty members, of course, may have received salary from no other source or from any one or a combination of four additional sources, as tabulated in Table 6-4. Of these other sources, the largest (Clin) was clinical professional fees, which paid a total of $246M in salary to 1,064 sponsored faculty, accounting for 51% of the salary they earned; this subgroup earned 32% of its income from sponsored sources (Table 6-4). A smaller number of sponsored faculty, 564, received some amount of "instructional" income, paid from the State Educational Appropriation; their instructional or sponsored income accounted (on average) for 27% or 44% of their salary, respectively. Gifts, endowments, and other sources contributed relatively little salary to smaller numbers of sponsored faculty (Table 6-4).

Faculty members receive different proportions of sponsored salary. At research-intensive medical schools in the US, faculty researchers reportedly receive about 50% of their salary from sponsored sources (11). At UCSF, the overall per-

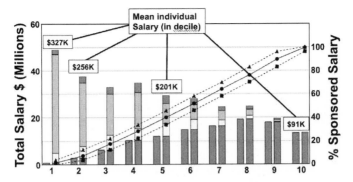

Fig. 6-1. Sources of salary for research faculty (those who received some salary from sponsored research). Each pair of columns (moving from left to right) represents a single decile of the 1,498 UCSF faculty who received some dollars in salary from a sponsored source in FY2014 (*10*). Deciles (numbered 1-10) are arranged in order of increasing percentage, from left to right, of total salary earned from a sponsoring source. For each decile, the column on the left represents the millions of dollars ($M; scale at far left) in sponsored salary (Spons $) earned, while the height of the column on the right represents the total salary dollars ($M, scale at far left) earned from all sources. Segments within each rightward column indicate the relative $M (scale at far left) earned by that decile from various sources, including (from bottom to top): sponsored dolllars; state educational funds; clinical revenues; gifts and endowments; other. Diagonal lines rising from left to right indicate the mean (circles), maximum (triangles), or minimum (squares) of sponsored dollars for each decile, as percentages of total salary, indicated on the scale at the far right. Black numbers above deciles 1, 2, 5, and 10 represent the mean total yearly salary of individuals in those deciles; the average salary was calculated by dividing the total $M for that decile by the number of individuals in that decile. Because the 1,498 faculty represented could not be evenly divided by 10, two deciles (numbers 5 and 10) contained 149 individual faculty; the other deciles contained 150 faculty.

centage is lower: the 1,498 faculty who receive some salary from sponsored sources receive, on average, 38% of salary from such sources, but averages like these can hide instructive heterogeneity. At UCSF this is very much the case, as shown by dividing sponsored faculty into deciles ranked by the proportions of sponsored salary in each decile (Figs. 6-1 to 6-3). Each decile includes 150 or 149 faculty members (Fig. 6-1 legend). In all three figures, the ten faculty deciles (numbered 1-10) are arranged in order of increasing proportions of sponsored income, from left to right; those proportions are indicated by diagonal lines that rise from the left, showing mean, maximum, and minimum % sponsored salary in each decile (quantified in the ordinate at the right of in Figs. 6-1 to 6-3). In these figures, each decile shows a pair of columns, whose heights correspond to millions of dollars in salary (left-hand scale) received by that decile; the leftward column of each pair represents sponsored salary, while the rightward column represents total salary dollars paid from UCSF

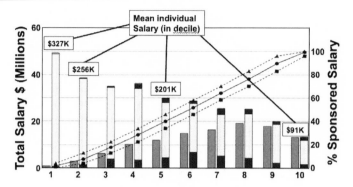

Fig. 6-2. Departments of research faculty (those who received some salary from sponsored research). Each pair of columns (moving from left to right) represents a single decile of the 1,498 UCSF faculty who received some dollars in salary from a sponsored source in FY2014 (*10*). With the single exception of the segments shown in the rightward column corresponding to each decile (for which, see below), all other aspects of this figure are identical to the same aspects in Fig. 6-1, including: scales at far left and far right; order and arrangement of deciles; heights and meaning of the leftward column in each decile; actual total height of the rightward column in each decile; diagonal lines rising from left to right; dollars of average annual salary (e.g., $327K) for deciles 1, 2, 5, and 10. For each decile, segments within each rightward column indicate the relative $M earned by faculty in that decile who belong to different kinds of academic department (*8*), including (from bottom to top): basic science; clinical; Organized Research Units; Other. Note that Organized Research Units are not present in decile 1, and the rather small "other" category is completely absent from deciles 2, 3, 6, and 8-10.

sources to members of that decile and contains bands whose meanings (and sizes) differ in Figs. 6-1 to 6-3. Together, these column pairs tell a pair of intertwined, intriguing stories.

Let us begin with Fig. 6-1. Note that in this and the other two figures the total salary dollars received by deciles (and thus mean total annual salary of the deciles' faculty) decrease markedly as % sponsored salary increases: faculty members who receive the highest annual salary (a mean of $327,000 per person for decile 1) receive less than 1%, on average, of their income from sponsored sources; at the scale's other end, decile 10's faculty receive nearly all their pay from sponsored funds, for a mean of $91,000 per year, or ~28% of the mean yearly salary of colleagues in decile 1. In an institution that reveres research, faculty whose incomes depend almost entirely on sponsored research receive far less total income than their richer colleagues. In a moment, we shall return to this striking irony.

A second story told in Fig. 6-1 is subtler, but still comes as a surprise to many academics. Although the average sponsored faculty member at UCSF

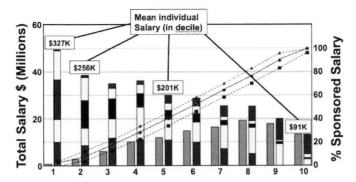

Fig. 6-3. Faculty series of research faculty (those who received some salary from sponsored research). Each pair of columns (moving from left to right) represents a single decile of the 1,498 UCSF faculty who received some dollars in salary from a sponsored source in FY2014 (*10*). With the single exception of the segments shown in the rightward column corresponding to each decile (for which, see below), all other aspects of this figure are identical to the same aspects in Fig. 6-1, including: scales at far left and far right; order and arrangement of deciles; heights and meaning of the leftward column in each decile; actual total height of the rightward column in each decile; diagonal lines rising from left to right; dollars of average annual salary (e.g., $327K) in deciles 1, 2, 5, and 10. For each decile, segments within each rightward column indicate the relative $M (scale at far left) earned by faculty in that decile who are appointed in each of five different faculty series (from bottom to top): ladder rank (absent in deciles 9 and 10); in residence; professor of clinical X; health science clinical; Adjunct.

received only 38% of her/his salary from sponsored sources (Table 6-1), half of UCSF's $114M in sponsored salary went to about one third of its sponsored faculty, each of whom received 65% or more of her/his salary from sponsored projects. (This one third are faculty in the 3.3 deciles toward the right of the graph.) The remaining half ($57M) of sponsored dollars went to the other 67% of sponsored faculty. This is no paradox: the bulk of sponsored salary must go to faculty who receive higher proportions of their salary from sponsoring sources. Still, the former dean of a large, research-intensive medical school (not UCSF) told one of the authors he was certain that not one of his research faculty received anywhere near 100% salary from grants, because sponsored research provides, on average, only about half a researcher's salary. The latter assertion may have been correct (*11*), but the first was almost surely wrong. Like an optical illusion, knowing that the average sponsored researcher at UCSF receives ~38% of her/his salary from sponsored sources encourages the illusory inference that most faculty members receive similar proportions of salary from grants. Instead, the deciles show that a substantial subset of

UCSF faculty researchers receives most of its salary from sources over which the host institution has no little or no control.

What do the deciles really tell us? Examining the different non-sponsored funds these faculty receive and how they distribute among different department types, academic ranks, and faculty series (Figures 6-1 to 6-3) tells a more complex tale, which interweaves the inverse correlation between total annual salary and % sponsored salary with the blunted perception of the highly leveraged salaries of research faculty. Thus segments in the taller right-hand column of each decile's pair in Fig. 6-1 show how the salary dollars received by that decile are distributed among different salary sources. The proportion of sponsored salary increases from left to right: in deciles 1-4 (with proportionally lower sponsored salary, on the left), three other salary sources predominate: clinical revenue (Clin); a smaller contribution from the State Education Appropriation (Instructional); and an even smaller amount from gifts and endowments (G&E); in deciles 5-10, these latter segments progressively decrease in size, as they are replaced by sponsored salary.

Fig. 6-2 shows how total salary dollars in different deciles distribute among different types of academic departments. Because most (82%; Table 6-3) of UCSF's sponsored faculty are located in clinical departments, by far the most total salary dollars in every decile go to clinical faculty. Most salary received by researchers in basic science departments falls into the middle deciles of sponsored faculty (deciles 3-8)—that is, the deciles in which faculty receive between 20 and 75% of salary from sponsoring sources. The basic vs. clinical differences reflect two circumstances. First, relative absence of basic science faculty from the first two deciles (high total salaries, low proportions of sponsored salary) reflects the inability of PhDs to supplement meager grant funds with clinical revenues. Second, basic science faculty are scarce in deciles 9 and 10 because, as we noted earlier, the historical dependence of basic science researchers on generous salary support from the university produced a culture in which young scientists are unwilling to be recruited without such support and established faculty insist on receiving it, despite dramatic reductions in the tax dollars needed to maintain it. For faculty in Organized Research Units, the decile distributions of salaries do not support strong inferences, because the numbers are too small.

As might be expected, age and academic rank also vary among the deciles (data not shown): assistant professors predominate in deciles 8-10, full professors in the more highly remunerated first four deciles; associate professors distribute more evenly among deciles.

So far, we can infer that: (i) clinical income and (to a much lower extent) state instructional funds account for most of the salaries paid to sponsored faculty who receive 50% or less of their salary from sponsored projects; (ii) most faculty in all deciles are members of clinical departments, but basic science department faculty tend to accumulate in the middle deciles, with sponsored salaries between 20% and 75% of total salary; (iii) faculty with the highest total salaries tend to receive most of their salary from clinical revenues (i.e., in deciles 1-4), with relatively small amounts from sponsored sources, while faculty with lower total salaries tend to receive fewer dollars from clinical sources (even though they belong to clinical departments), and earn very high proportions of salary from sponsored sources.

Fig. 6-3 shows how dollars paid to faculty in the five different faculty series distribute among faculty deciles sorted according to proportion of sponsored salary. We might expect nuanced distributions of faculty series among these deciles, because membership in each series is supposed to specify both coveted privileges (e.g., sabbatical leave or voting in the Academic Senate) and how UCSF judges a faculty member for promotion. Two trends stand out. First, faculty with less than 80% of salary supplied from sponsored sources (deciles 1-7) tend to belong predominantly to one of three faculty series: (i) *the ladder rank series*, probably because this series includes many highly respected (and highly remunerated) members of clinical departments, who are expected to contribute equally in research and teaching; (ii) perhaps for similar reasons, earnings of the *in residence* series also group toward the left side, although this series extends more widely into deciles 8 and 9 as well; (iii) the *professor of clinical X* series probably distributes toward the left side because they can earn substantial salaries from clinical service and because research prowess is not as strong a requirement for their promotion. Second, the adjunct series is distributed mostly into deciles 7-10, which earn high proportions of sponsored salaries, in keeping with the fact that an adjunct faculty member can be promoted on the basis of excellence in research or teaching, but equal contributions in both areas are not required (Table 6-2).

Fig. 6-3 contains two mysterious surprises. The first is decile 1, in which 150 sponsored faculty appear to receive less than $1M in total sponsored salary but earn (on average) very large salaries. One suspects that their researcher status is largely honorary, and that few of these well remunerated individuals seriously engage in research. Still, the apparition of 150 ghostly researchers in honorary lab coats—along with ~$50M earned from non-sponsored sources (Fig. 6-1)—probably explains why the overall population of UCSF's sponsored researchers garner on average only 38% of their salaries from sponsored sources; in contrast, the ~50% average (*11*) at other research universities suggests their non-researchers find honorary lab coats less attractive. A second mysterious surprise is the low average salary ($91,000) of faculty in decile 10. Some may be part-time employees; full-time employment is not required for adjunct faculty, who predominate in this decile.

Perspective

In FY2014, soft-money salaries paid ~38% of all UCSF faculty researchers' salary, and ~21% of all faculty salary, but many researchers receive very large fractions of their salary from grants. Their resulting vulnerability to slight downturns in external funding makes them less likely to promote innovative discovery, and heavy reliance on soft money salaries for those researchers may weaken UCSF's willingness to apply its own standards to judge the quality of research, at a time when that quality is severely threatened by external economic forces. Subsequent chapters will return to these issues.

Chapter 7

Put money in thy (research) purse: Funds, administration, and goals

In previous chapters we began to see how multiple external pressures test and re-test UCSF's ability to accomplish its research mission. Here and in subsequent chapters, our focus shifts to examining how UCSF's internal environment shapes goals and day-to-day conduct of research in labs, research groups, and departments. In addition to competing institutional missions, the research effort's *milieu intérieur* includes a formidable array of schools, departments and other administrative entities; dense thickets of academic rules, regulations, and customs; diverse funding models awash in acronyms, competition, and occasional mystery; changing standards of scientific value; and tightly woven webs of dollars and programs designed to train young scientists.

This chapter describes the different types of academic units—clinical departments and non-clinical departments, which include basic science departments, social science departments, and "Organized Research Units" (ORUs)—that administer UCSF's research. Here we sketch histories of these types, compare their scopes, relative sizes, and funding, and set the stage for focusing on basic and social science departments and ORUs (chapter 8) and on clinical departments (chapter 9). Chapter 10 weighs answers to large questions posed in chapters 7, 8 and 9.

A short history

For many decades, a troublesome fault line has zigzagged through most US medical schools, separating their faculty into either of two department types: clinical, which teach medical students and resident physicians how to diagnose and treat disease, and non-clinical sciences—originally grouped under the rubric of "basic" sciences—which teach human biology and pathogenesis. Through the 20th century, clinical and basic science professors sometimes worked together, but also competed—sometimes fiercely. When a geological fault line produced the devastating 1906 earthquake in San Francisco, the "UC Medical School" split in two, geographically and pedagogically: first-year students were taught anatomy, physiology, and pathology in Berkeley, and transferred across the Bay to the Parnassus campus the next year, to learn clinical medicine. For fifty years, Berkeley's academic ethos encouraged the medical school's pre-clinical science faculty to take pride in "pure" research, unblemished by any need to produce useful results. Meanwhile, their clinical colleagues across the Bay criticized basic research as not relevant to patients and disease (1). UC finally brought pre-clinical departments and their students back to San Francisco in 1958, when the UC Medical School combined with other schools to become UCSF. An illustrious basic science faculty member, who elected to stay in Berkeley, characterized UCSF's new 14-story hospital as a "skyscraper exclusively inhabited by pygmies" (2). Emphatically disagreeing, UCSF's clinicians and its chancellor staunchly followed the banner of teaching and practicing clinical medicine, and many feared that growing NIH largesse and "rat-doctors" would divert precious university resources to research (1).

In 1964, a formidable delegation of UCSF faculty triggered a decisive directional shift, by requesting that UC's president, Clark Kerr, find a replacement for their chancellor, John Saunders—who, they argued, would never foster the outstanding research required of a leading academic biomedical center. Sharing their hopes for UCSF, Kerr made his own inquiries, and deftly replaced Saunders in 1965. This academic coup depended on crucial but surprising support from chairs of five *clinical* departments, who acted in coalition with the medical school dean and a visionary physiologist who headed the Cardiovascular Research Institute (CVRI; 3), which was to become UCSF's first and most successful Organized Research Unit, or ORU. (ORUs are academic units of UC whose principal function is research, within a specifically targeted area; see 4.) That clinical support was made possible by the dean's recent recruitments (unopposed and perhaps undetected by Saunders) of clinical department chairs from first-rate research-intensive east coast schools. Their presence in the delegation to UC's leader made it clear that a campus that failed to support research would not long retain ambitious, forward-thinking clinician-scholars (1, 4, 5).

Indeed, the coup did produce important consequences for research at UCSF, initially by freeing up new laboratory space in towers constructed with UC dollars and bringing bright new researchers to clinical departments. By the end of the 1960s, these researchers, along with others in the CVRI, began to attract enough NIH dollars to match those of leading east coast medical

Table 7-1. UCSF: Contributions and Discoveries

Contribution**	Contributor	Year
1999 or before		
Editor, *Science* magazine	Bruce Alberts	2008-13
Director, National Institutes of Health	Harold Varmus	1993-99
Asst Secretary for Health, Health & Human Services Dept*	Philip R. Lee	1965-69
FDA Commissioner	Jere Goyan	1979-81
2000-2015		
Council, Institute of Medicine	Nancy Adler	2010-
President, National Academy of Science	Bruce Alberts	1993-2005
CEO, Bill and Melinda Gates Foundation*	Susan Desmond-Hellman	2014-
Director, Center for Disease Control	Julie Gerberding	2002-9
Advisory Council to NIH Director	Keith Yamamoto	2004-10
Chair, Coalition for the Life Sciences		2006-12
Vice President, CSO, HHMI*	Erin O'Shea	2013-
Director, National Cancer Institute	Harold Varmus	2010-15

Major Discoveries**	Discoverer	
Oncogenes	Michael Bishop, Harold Varmus	1970s
Recombinant DNA technology	Herbert Boyer[¶]	1970s
Cloning of insulin gene in bacteria	William Rutter[§]	1970s
Prenatal tests for sickle cell anemia and thalassemia	Y.W. Kan	1970
Pharmacists as drug therapy specialists	School of Pharmacy	1970s
Prions	Stanley Prusiner	1980s
First academic hospitalist program	Robert Wachter	1990s
Telomerase, telomere biology	Elizabeth Blackburn[‡]	1980s
Catheter ablation therapy for tachycardia	Melvin Scheinman	1980s
Pluripotent stem cells made from skin cells	Shinya Yamanaka	2000s

*Abbreviations: Asst, assistant; CEO, Chief Executive Officer; CSO, Chief Scientific Officer; HHMI, Howard Hughes Medical Institute
¶With Stanley Cohen, Stanford University.
§With UCSF colleagues.
‡Telomerase was co-discovered with Carol Greider.
**This table's information was compiled as described in reference 9.

schools, Johns Hopkins and Columbia (6)—an impressive "catch-up" feat for a late arrival to the federal research banquet. The coup also allowed the medical school dean, working with the chair of medicine in 1969, to recruit William Rutter to the chair of Biochemistry, where he fashioned a pattern that later extended to other basic science departments (7).

In the 1970s and 1980s, UCSF produced four remarkable and surprising discoveries: development of recombinant DNA technology; the first oncogene, *src*; a new class of infectious agent, the prion, which transmits Creuzfeldt-Jakob disease; and founding of the first successful biotechnology company, Genentech (*8*). Each surprise transformed biomedical research and much of clinical medicine, world-wide.

Since the 1970s, UCSF faculty made major contributions to biomedicine and many discoveries (Table 7-1; *9*). While the four surprises did not directly result from the 1964 coup or from Rutter's recruitment, in combination they exerted important effects:

1. Research in UCSF's basic science departments rapidly accelerated, owing both to the DNA-based revolution in biological research and to the fact that three of the four surprises of the 1970s-1980s originated in basic science departments (*8*). Following Biochemistry's lead and strongly supported by the institution, in the 1980s these departments recruited new chairs and exciting scientists, created an innovative coalition of graduate programs, and produced superb science, recognized by multiple honors, including prestigious Lasker, Shaw, and Nobel prizes (Table 7-2; *9*).

2. Combined with the DNA revolution, the success of Genentech and other biotechnology companies kindled entrepreneurial research at UCSF and many other biomedical research centers, in both clinical and basic science departments.

3. In 2003 UCSF moved many basic science faculty to the new campus at Mission Bay. Their new quarters distanced them from clinical faculty at Parnassus, and not only geographically: clinician-scientists began wondering why—despite outnumbering the departees and garnering more sponsored research dollars—they seemed to attract less of UCSF's attention and remained in cramped, less lavish laboratories.

Over time, the ascendancy of basic science research increased UCSF's prestige and attracted more excellent scientists to UCSF, to join clinical and other departments. These and other influences gradually promoted growth and increased power of clinical departments. A key part of UCSF's research story stems from this new ascendancy.

In the meantime, UCSF's research continues to make widely recognized contributions to biomedical science. Table 7-2 emphasizes awards and honors in the 21st century: in 2014 UCSF had 18 Howard Hughes Medical Institute (HHMI) Investigators; since 2000, 17 UCSF faculty were elected into the National Academy of Sciences, six received awards that often precede the Nobel—including four Lasker Awards, one Passano Award, and five Shaw

Table 7-2. Science Awards to
UCSF Faculty, 2001-present*

Award	Year	Department
HHMI Investigators[¶] (18 in 2014)		Basic science 14; clinical 4
Gairdner Award		
Six awards, 1984-1993		
Peter Walter	2009	Biochemistry and Biophysics
Shinya Yamanaka	2009	Anatomy
Lasker Award		
(Eight awards, 1951-1994)		
Elizabeth Blackburn	2006	Biochemistry and Biophysics
Shinya Yamanaka	2009	Anatomy, Gladstone Institutes
Ronald Vale	2012	Cell. and Molec. Pharmacology
Peter Walter	2014	Biochemistry
National Academy of Sciences		
>30 before 1999		
Seventeen, 2000-present		Basic science 14; clinical 3
National Medal of Science		
Bruce Alberts	2014	Biochemistry and Biophysics
National Medal of Science &		
Technology		
(One before 2000)		
Harold Varmus	2001	Microbiology and Immunology
Michael Bishop	2003	Microbiology and Immunology
Stanley Prusiner	2011	Neurology
Nobel Laureates		
(Three, 1984-1997)		
Elizabeth Blackburn	2009	Biochemistry and Biophysics
Shinya Yamanaka	2012	Anatomy, Gladstone Institutes
Passano Award		
(Four before 2000)		
David Julius	2010	Physiology
Shaw Prize		
YW Kan	2004	Medicine
Herbert Boyer	2004	Biochemistry and Biophysics
Shinya Yamanaka	2008	Anatomy
David Julius	2010	Physiology
Peter Walter	2014	Biochemistry and Biophysics

*Award information was compiled as described in reference 9.
¶Abbreviation: HHMI, Howard Hughes Medical Institute

Prizes—and two did receive Nobel prizes.

Before we proceed further, it is important not to conflate classifications of research as "clinical" vs. "basic" in scope, methods, and goals with its classification as conducted, housed, and funded in clinical departments vs. basic science departments and ORUs. Years ago, the classification of research may have accorded more closely with the type of department, but walls do not easily confine scientific curiosity. In fact many researchers in clinical departments seek to answer "basic" questions focused on underlying mechanisms, biological and otherwise—just as researchers in basic science departments and ORUs often delight in questions regarding the pathogenesis and therapy of disease.

Table 7-3. Sponsored salary and sponsored Revenue in FY2014, by department type*

Department type[‖]:		Basic	ORUs	Basic + ORUs	Clinical	All depts
Sponsored faculty[§]	No.	197	78	275	1223	1498
Total salary	$M	34	14	48	254	30
Avge** total salary	$K	173	179	175	208	202
Sponsored salary	$M	17	7.8	25	89	114
Avge spons. sal.	$K	88	100	90	73	68
Spons./total sal.	%	51	56	52	35	38
Research C&G	$M	115	80	195	595	790
(TDC)[‡] Avge/spons. fac.	$K	584	1,030	—	487	527
Indirect cost (IC)[‡] rec.	$M	42	31	73	125	198
	$K	212	397	—	102	132
Avge/spons. fac. TDC + IC	$M	157	111	268	720	988
(TDC+IC)/spons. fac.	$K	797	1,423	—	588	659

*Data represents all UCSF's schools and departments in FY2014, but excludes faculty who received no salary from any sponsored research project. Numbers of sponsored faculty are not identical with those of PIs on sponsored projects, because some faculty receive salary only from research dollars awarded to another faculty member.

¶UCSF's schools include 12 basic science departments, seven ORUs, and 26 clinical departments (10).

§Numbers of faculty with primary appointments in the different department types and their total and sponsored salaries are as shown in chapter 6, Table 6-3, except that the present table combines ORUs with the very much smaller "other" category. Note: all salary figures pertain to faculty who received sponsored salary; salaries paid to non-faculty personnel from sponsored project funds are not included.

‡TDC and IC of contracts and grants are in (11).

**Abbreviations: avge, average; C&G, contracts and grants; fac., faculty; IC, indirect cost; rec., recovered; spons, sponsored; $M, millions of dollars; $K, thousands of dollars; ORU, Organized Research Unit, such as the Cardiovascular Research Institute; sal., salary; TDC, total direct cost.

In this and the next two chapters we focus primarily on research similarities and differences between different department types, but we shall also point out differences—which may exist within individual departments and department types—that relate to the basic vs. clinical scope of the research itself. Traditional department types and the geographic separation of researchers in those types may pose important questions for guiding UCSF's future research, to be discussed in subsequent chapters.

Research in department types: quantitative comparisons

This section will examine numbers of sponsored faculty and their salaries, research funding, and research space in different department types. Tables 7-3 and 7-4 present FY2014 data from UCSF's four Schools, with their total of 26 clinical departments, 12 non-clinical departments broadly defined as "basic science," and seven ORUs (*4, 10*).

Clinical department faculty researchers greatly outnumber researchers in other department types (Table 7-3). The 1,223 clinical department faculty who receive some portion of their salary from sponsored research contracts and grants are ~6-fold more numerous than their sponsored colleagues in basic science departments and ~4-fold more numerous than the 275 sponsored faculty in basic science departments and ORUs combined. Total research funding in clinical departments ($720M = total direct costs + indirect costs) is also several-fold greater than in either basic science departments or the combination of basic science and ORUs. Compared to the headcount difference, the funding difference is less marked: for clinical vs. (basic + ORU) the funding ratio is 2.7 while the headcount ratio is 4.5. The difference reflects two differences between research grants and contracts in clinical vs. other UCSF departments: (i) per capita, sponsored faculty in basic science departments or ORUs receive larger ($584K or $1,030K, respectively) total direct costs (TDC) in grants and contract dollars than do sponsored clinical faculty ($487K); (ii) indirect cost recovery (here termed ICR* because it is calculated as a % of TDC, rather than MTDC; see chapter 6) is higher in basic science or ORUs (ICR* = 36% or 39%, respectively), compared to clinical departments (ICR* = 21%); in turn, these differences reflect the fact that a larger proportion of clinical department contracts and grants comes from non-federal (private) sources, which usually pay indirect costs—when they do so at all—at much lower rates than does the NIH. So far, the comparisons in Table 7-3 support straightforward inferences.

1. As a group, clinical departments have many more sponsored faculty and bring in substantially larger numbers of sponsored dollars than non-clinical departments.
2. The average sponsored faculty member in a clinical department attracts fewer research dollars than her/his colleagues in other departments, and the average basic science researcher brings in fewer grant dollars than the average ORU researcher; these differences may reflect, at least in part, the relative time and effort "average" faculty members in each of

Table 7-4. Sponsored salary, sponsored revenue, and research space, by department type*

Department type[||]:		Basic	ORUs	Clinical	All depts
Sponsored faculty[§]	No.	197	78	1223	1498
TDC + IC**[§]	$M	157	111	720	988
Research space[#]	Sq.ft (K)	412	241	937	1,590
Ratios					
Space/spons. fac	Sq.ft (K)	2,091	3,090	766	1,061
(TDC+IC)/spons. fac.	$K	797	1,423	588	659
(TDC+IC)/sq. ft.	$	381	461	771	621

*Data represents all UCSF's schools and departments in FY2014, but excludes faculty who received no salary from any sponsored research project. Numbers of sponsored faculty are not identical with those of PIs on sponsored projects, because a few faculty members do not serve as PIs of a grant or contract, but nonetheless receive salary from research dollars awarded to another faculty member.

[||]Together UCSF's schools include 12 basic science departments, seven ORUs, and 26 clinical departments (10).

[§]Exactly as described in the legend of Table 7-3.

[‡]TDC and IC of contracts and grants are in reference 11.

[#]Research space is tabulated in reference 12.

**Abbreviations: avge, average; fac., faculty; IC, indirect cost; rec., recovered; spons, sponsored; $M, millions of dollars; K, thousands, $K, thousands of dollars; ORU, Organized Research Unit, such as the Cardiovascular Research Institute; Sq. ft., square feet; TDC, total direct cost.

these units devote to research.

3. The difference is even greater if we compare only indirect costs per sponsored faculty member: $212,000 or $397,000 per basic science or ORU researcher, respectively, vs. $102,000 per average clinical researcher (Table 7-3).

In summary, average individual researchers in clinical departments attract fewer direct cost dollars, and recovery of indirect costs on their sponsored research pays lower proportions of the associated indirect costs incurred by the university. We shall ask in a moment what these differences may mean for UCSF's overall research effort.

One source of smoldering contention relates to a third difference between clinical and basic science departments—that is, the disproportionate greater research space available to basic scientists and ORUs (mostly on the Mission Bay campus), relative to space available to researchers in clinical departments (mostly on the Parnassus campus). In raw numbers, the disparity is real (Table 7-4): the average sponsored faculty member in basic science departments and ORUs "owns" 2,091 and 3,090 assignable square feet, respectively, while the average sponsored clinical faculty researcher "owns" 766 assignable square feet, or ~3- to 4-fold less. But researchers in clinical departments can devote (on average) less time and effort to research, so it may be useful to compare the research "earnings" (TDC + IC) of the average square foot of research space. Calculated in this way (Table 7-4), in FY2014 the average square foot of research space in basic science departments or ORUs garnered, respectively, $381 or $461 in sponsored dollars (TDC + IC), while the average square foot of clinical research space garnered $771 such dollars—nearly twice as much.

Although quantitatively impressive, these differences may also mislead, owing to specific aspects of the space required for some kinds of research in clinical departments: (i) a clinical trial may be performed (mostly) in space that belongs to the medical enterprise and formally not "research space" at all; (ii) certain research with living patients is not performed in clinical space, but must be rented by researchers in departments and divisions; (iii) patient-focused research (e.g., studies of clinical outcomes, implementation of alternative diagnostic or therapeutic regimens, analysis of biomarkers in patient populations, etc.) often requires mostly "dry-lab" space (where researchers work with computers, desks, and files, and little or no "wet-lab" space like that in basic science departments and many ORUs. Analysts at UCSF and elsewhere have not accurately quantitated proportions of dry-lab, wet-lab, hospital-furnished, and rented clinical research space in any departments. So, we don't know whether, or to what extent, the apparent space-crunch reflects wet labs smaller than their basic science department counterparts, a plethora of dry-lab research and space, research in clinics and wards not defined as research space, research with patients in space the clinical enterprise cannot provide, or, most likely, a combination of all these possibilities.

Thus the clinical department space crunch is probably real, but it is premature to "fix" it without thinking hard about the actual value, for the institution, of different kinds of research space. Imagine that UCSF magically knew, to the square inch, the size of every kind of research space imaginable, in every department, throughout the institution—what should UCSF do with that information? We encounter yet another confounding example of the Muddlement Uncertainty Principle (M-UP). One way or another, UCSF and other institutions will have to work out (or blindly decide) how to compare values of

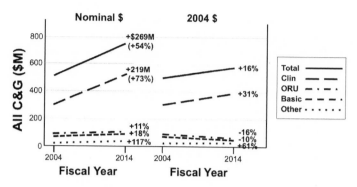

Fig. 7-1. Changes in sponsored research funds, FY2004 vs. FY2014: All Contracts and Grants (C&G). Values are graphed in nominal dollars (left panel) or 2004 dollars (right panel); in each panel, numbers to the right show dollars in FY2014 and percentage change relative to FY2004. Lines connect the 2004 and 2014 values for (in order, from top to bottom of each panel) Total dollars, and those awarded to different department types: Clinical, ORU, Basic Science (Basic), or Other.

different kinds of space (*13*). While it will be fascinating to see how these co-nundrums are resolved, we remind readers that the Executive Vice Chancellor has already issued a *quantitative* requirement that research units must recover indirect costs of $90/asf, a value that will increase to $120/asf in 2016. We refer readers to chapter 4, where we argued that charging ICR dollars as rent is an unfortunate and misguided approach. Instead, UCSF must gather better data and define the values of different kinds of research with genuine care and clarity.

Clinical department research grows faster

Although the actual numbers are hard to pin down, clinician researchers al-most surely outnumbered basic scientists at UCSF in the early 1970s, and clini-cal departments also garnered more NIH grant dollars—and probably con-tinued to do so through the rest of the 20th century. What about the critical 11 fiscal years from 2004 to 2014? Congress doubled NIH's budget between 1999 and 2003, but a severe recession and Congressional gridlock decisively damped the budget's growth for the next 11 years. The disastrous result : in inflation-corrected dollars (*14*), NIH had 21% less to spend in FY 2014 than in FY2004. (In nominal dollars, the NIH budget in 2014 was $29.9B, barely 6.7% greater than in 2004.)

Within UCSF, we shall focus on growth of research in the School of

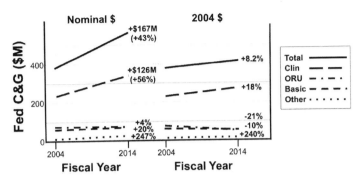

Fig. 7-2. Changes in sponsored federal research funds, FY2004 vs. FY2014. Values are graphed in nominal dollars (left panel) or 2004 dollars (right panel); in each panel, numbers to the right show dollars in FY2014 and percentage change relative to FY2004. Lines connect the 2004 and 2014 values for (in order, from top to bottom of each panel) Total dollars, and those awarded to different department types: Clinical, ORU, Basic Science (Basic), or Other.

Medicine, which hosts by far the largest number of researchers and garners most of UCSF's grant money. In this School, rivalry between clinical and non-clinical departments is especially keen. Compare three measures of the medical school's sponsored research dollars in 2004 vs. 2014 (*11, 15*): total research dollars (Fig. 7-1), federal research dollars (Fig. 7-2), and private, non-federal research dollars (Fig. 7-3). In each Figure, the dollars represent the sum of total direct costs plus indirect costs, either in nominal dollars (on the left) or inflation-corrected, 2004 dollars (on the right). First, consider the relative sizes of all research funds garnered by different department types in 2004, when clinical departments received $301M in total sponsored research, or 60% of the School's entire $500M in sponsored research (*17*). Other department types garnered fewer dollars: $87M (17% of the total) for basic sciences; $96M (19%) for ORUs, and $18M (3.6%) for units in the "other" category. Federally sponsored research awards ($387M) to different department types showed a similar pattern. From private, non-federal sources, UCSF received $113M, with clinical departments garnering the lion's share ($81M; 72%).

How did the different department types fare in FY2014, as compared to 2004? In nominal dollars, total sponsored research funds in 2014 ($769M) exceeded the 2004 total by $269M, or 54% (Fig. 7-1, left panel). Four fifths (81%) of the increase reflects the $219M (73%) increase in research funds received by clinical departments. Basic science and ORUs showed lower percentage gains (18 and 11%, respectively); for this reason, and because they

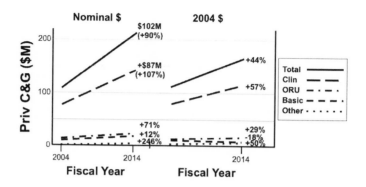

Fig. 7-3. Changes in sponsored research funds from private (Priv) sources, FY2004 vs. FY2014. Values are graphed in nominal dollars (left panel) or 2004 dollars (right panel); in each panel, numbers to the right show dollars in FY2014 and percentage change relative to FY2004. Lines connect the 2004 and 2014 values for (in order, from top to bottom of each panel) Total dollars, and those awarded to different department types: Clinical, ORU, Basic Science (Basic), or Other.

started at a lower level in 2004, in 2014 their contributions to the large increase in the school's overall sponsored research dollars were not impressive. [The tiny "other" category grew rapidly (+117% in 11 years), but started at such a low level that its contribution to the overall picture was small.]

It is instructive to compare changes in the school's federal vs. its private (non-federal) sponsored research from 2004 to 2014. In nominal dollars (left panels of Figs. 7-2 and 3), overall federal C&G rose by $167M (+43%: Fig. 7-2), while private research rose by $102M—less in absolute terms, but proportionately more than twice as fast (90% increase; Fig. 7-3). For both funding sources, the bulk of the overall increase took place in clinical departments: a 56% rise in federal funding for these departments accounted for three fourths of the overall federal increase, while their 107% increase in private research funds accounted for 85% of the overall growth in private funding. Contributions of basic science departments and ORUs to the growth in overall grant revenues were diminished both by their relatively low percentage increases in federal grant dollars and also by the comparatively low proportions of total grant dollars awarded to these department types by private funders (Figs. 7-2 and 7-3, left panels).

All in all, the medical school fared well in a period that saw less than 7% cumulative growth in NIH's budget, in nominal dollars. But correcting dollar values of research funds accrued in 2014 for inflation during the past 11 years (right-hand panels of Figs 7-1 to 7-3) presents a more realistic and sobering story. In inflation-corrected dollars, the School's federal research funds increased by 8.2%, while NIH budgets fell by 21% (Fig. 2); in part owing to a 44% increase in private research funding (Fig. 7-3), the School's overall research funding rose by 16% (in 2004 dollars; Fig. 7-1). In sharp contrast to the 31% overall increase for clinical departments, however, basic science departments and ORUs experienced 10 and 16% reductions, respectively, in overall research funding (Fig. 7-1, 2004 dollars); although ORUs managed to increase their private research funding by 29%, private funding for basic science departments decreased by 21%—both changes were dwarfed by the 57% increase for clinical departments (inflation-corrected dollars, Fig. 7-3, right panel).

Now compare these changes with changes in revenues of UCSF's campus and its clinical enterprise: from 2004 to 2014, inflation-corrected revenues of the clinical enterprise rose by 58%, total campus revenues by only 20% (*17*). Two correlations are striking: (i) clinical enterprise revenues and the medical school's research funds from private (non-federal) sources rose by high (58% vs. 44%) margins; (ii) similarly, inflation-corrected growth of the School's overall research funds and that of campus revenues were both low (16 and 20%, respectively). Anti-correlations to the parallel prosperity of clinical departments and the clinical enterprise are equally striking: basic science and ORU research funds both decreased substantially during the same period (Fig. 7-1, right panel). Correlations do not prove causation, but these correlations strongly suggest two tentative inferences, which may be correct: (i) clinical departments successfully attracted private funds in parallel with continued prosperity of the clinical enterprise itself; (ii) non-clinical departments and some ORUs had much less success in attracting private research funds because donors and companies considered their research less likely to benefit patients or increase profits of the medical care industry. Basic science researchers received more prizes and honors awards than their clinical counterparts, who instead garnered increasing support for their work.

Perspective

The histories of UCSF's different department types and quantitative comparisons of their present grant revenues and growth over the past 11 years reveal both encouraging success and disturbing hints of present and future difficulties. This chapter highlights issues that should concern researchers in both clinical and "basic" departments:

1. UCSF devotes immense resources to its research mission, with gratifying results in a 21st century barely 15 years old, as indicated by overall research funding, prizes and other accolades, and ability to attract excellent students and faculty.

2. The institution's research investments and accomplishments are even more impressive in view of the many serious economic and financial challenges during this period: decreases in state funds, stagnant federal research budgets, and stiffer competition from rich institutions with vast endowments, well-heeled alumni, and ability to attract generous philanthropy.

3. As UCSF's clinical enterprise prospered and grew in the 20th century, research in clinical departments became highly successful in attracting both federal and private research funds. Its research growth persisted through the past 11 years, even when economic stresses severely slowed growth of most academic research.

4. During this latter 11-year period, research in UCSF's basic science departments and ORUs suffered gradual but substantial reductions in overall research funding (corrected for inflation), and their research faculty and personnel did not increase. Compared to the 1990s, basic science departments find it more difficult to support faculty salaries and attract new faculty (see chapter 8).

5. Ignoring inflation blurs visions of both past and future. Nominal-dollar increases mask stark contrasts in research funding between clinical departments and basic science departments and ORUs, while inflation-corrected figures show why the latter researchers are discouraged: overall UCSF research triumphs over adversity, but their own resources continue to diminish. In a time of unparalleled research opportunity, their well-founded fear of falling behind is tinged with bitter irony.

Before we begin to focus more narrowly on research in the two major department types, differences between them raise important questions. First, related to causation: why did research funding rise in clinical departments between 2004 and 2014, but fall in ORUs and basic science departments (Fig. 7-1)? The second asks what to do: how should UCSF respond to the rising arc of one kind of research and decline of another?

It is by now means clear that UCSF has actually posed the what to do question in a deliberate, conscious fashion. But it may have already begun to answer hit, by unconsciously heeding the economic imperative of two paradoxes: compared to their colleagues in basic science departments and ORUs, individual researchers in clinical departments receive fewer research funds (in direct or indirect costs) and "own" considerably less research space; nonetheless, collectively the more numerous clinician-researchers garner ever-growing shares of UCSF's research dollars, so an average square foot of their research space accounts for almost twice as many research dollars as it does in their counterparts' laboratories. Rather than hire more basic scientists and build more laboratories, the university can attract more grant dollars by hiring many clinician-researchers, partly paid by the clinical enterprise, and investing less money for their laboratory space.

We suggest, in contrast, that UCSF should deliberately pose both questions and answer the second by judging the relative values of different kinds of research to the university, to its present and future researchers, and to ordinary citizens. These value judgments can prove critical for UCSF's future, as we shall see in chapter 10.

Chapter 8

Basic science departments:
The future ain't what it used to be

As chapter 7 showed, basic science departments and ORUs together garnered 29% of UCSF's sponsored research funding in FY2014, although their sponsored funding (corrected for inflation) had decreased 10-16% over the preceding 11 years. During the same period, in contrast, sponsored funding in clinical departments grew by 40%. If clinical departments find it so much easier to attract funds for studying diseases and new treatments, what is the present role of basic science departments within UCSF? In practical terms, research is the basic scientists' primary task, and determines their promotions and salaries; their teaching roles in medical or other professional schools have become much attenuated. A second question must be posed: what will or should be the proper role of basic science research at UCSF, 10 or 20 years hence?

This and subsequent chapters examine such questions, as they face researchers in both non-clinical and clinical departments. We describe research opportunities, strategies, and challenges of each department type in funding and guiding their investigators and in educating young scientists. Amid many similarities, these department types show striking differences.

Why don't basic scientists teach basic science to medical students?

This question relates directly to the present predicament of basic science department faculty at UCSF. Until the 1970s, their central function in UCSF's ecosystem was to teach "basic" human biology to professional students; their research focused on academic fields reflected in department names—anatomy, biochemistry, physiology, microbiology, and pharmacology. As research in basic science departments came to depend more on the fruits of the DNA

Table 8-1. Research in UCSF Basic Science Departments: 21st Century Examples

1. **Identifying the SARS virus** as a coronavirus (Joe Derisi; 2)
2. Finding **heat-detecting membrane receptors** and showing how they trigger heat-induced pain, in molecular detail (David Julius; 3)
3. Dissecting modular **neural control of sexually dimorphic behaviors** like mating, aggression, and pair bonding (Nirao Shah; 4)
4. Using 3D structures to devise **selective chemical inhibitors of kinases** that explain cell function and can treat disease (Kevan Shokat; 5)
5. Understanding molecular motors that move organelles and vesicles up and down microtubule highways to coordinate cell functions across distances varying from microns to a meter (Ronald Vale; 6)
6. Discovering how the **unfolded protein response** directs cells to build the factories that make all secreted proteins (Peter Walter; 7)
7. **Ribosome profiling** reveals in detail the specific spectrum of different proteins cells make at a particular moment (Jonathan Weissman; 8)

revolution, in the early 1980s, their research began to explore questions beyond old departmental confines, gradually achieved national prominence, and attracted generous NIH funding. Eager to focus more intently on research, young molecular and cell biologists preferred teaching graduate students (who would work in their labs), and their departments began to shift teaching responsibilities in professional courses to adjunct faculty PhDs. The new adjunct faculty became extremely good teachers—often better than the researchers who preceded them—and by the late 1980s assumed much greater roles in teaching and supervising professional courses. At first the basic science departments—then recipients of generous state support for faculty and administrative salaries and of more generous NIH grants—supplied substantial financial support for adjunct teaching faculty. As state support diminished and grants became harder to obtain, the medical school's contribution to salary support for adjunct teaching faculty progressively increased, but was still funneled through basic science departments.

By the 21st century, UCSF's medical school had begun a major shift of basic science teaching for medical students: away from traditional lectures and toward learning in small-group sessions focused at interfaces between "basic" knowledge and its application in the clinic. Pedagogically effective and by now predominant in the medical school, the new approach has been adopted by other schools (1). A cadre of 8-10 education-focused adjunct faculty, including several basic science department faculty hired more than two decades ago, plays a large role in planning and coordinating this new approach, and it appears to work well. It requires large numbers of teachers capable of teaching teach basic aspects of human biology and pathogenesis, integrated with clinical problem-solving. But medical school places less emphasis on basic human biology than in the 1980s, and UCSF's basic science researchers—well-versed in molecular biology and genetics—lack training in anatomy, pharmacology, physiology, microbiology, as well as clinical knowledge and skills. Although they still give a few lectures in professional courses, and/or teach small-group sections for medical students, their teaching focuses mostly on graduate students.

Bottom line: even if they wanted to, UCSF's basic science departments could never recapture their formerly un-replaceable status as teachers of health professionals. Thus the rationale for UCSF's support of basic science departments relies almost exclusively on the quality of their research.

Opportunities, goals, and diverse approaches

In basic science departments and ORUs, research targets range across broad expanses of biology, exemplified by Table 8-1's list of currently active projects. Like most basic science research projects, these share key elements:

1. Grounding in *molecular genetics*, structures of macromolecules, and how molecules work together in cells.
2. Primary *focus on mechanisms underlying critical life* processes, such as disease, pain, sex, functional diversity, and response to stress.
3. Work conducted in laboratories funded by public and private sources, in which PI faculty members direct efforts of graduate students and postdocs.
4. Intense collaboration with other labs in basic science or clinical departments at UCSF or other institutions.
5. Driven by curiosity about mechanisms, these projects also impinge, directly and indirectly, on devastating human diseases (projects 1 and 4), focus on processes that concern human welfare (projects 2 and 3), or explain fundamental life functions (5, 6 and 7) that are deranged in human disease.

The projects in Table 8-1 flourish in the second decade of the 21st century, owing to their PIs' imagination, drive, and scientific prowess. But those scientists' environment also made a huge difference. When they came to UCSF—three in the 1980s, three in the 1990s, one in 2003—they found able, welcoming, and interactive basic science colleagues, bright and vigorous graduate students and postdocs, and an administration eager to help them succeed. In 2003, they moved their laboratories into spacious new facilities on the new Mission Bay campus. They unite in emphasizing the significance for human welfare of fundamental research and its limitless opportunities in the 21st century. These opportunities "have never been brighter," says Jonathan Weissman (9). "New technologies provide unprecedented speed and depth, making studies of human tissues and cross-species comparisons vastly more powerful—especially at UCSF, with its ready access to technology, scientific talent, and patients."

In that context, we proceed to nitty-gritty quantitative facts about research in UCSF's non-clinical academic departments and ORUs (Table 8-2). UCSF moves back and forth between two general classifications of its non-clinical units. In one, adopted in earlier chapters of this book, these units are either ORUs or "basic science" departments. The second, which we use in the present chapter, separate "basic" from "social" science to come up with three headings: basic science, social science, and ORUs. Of 20 separate non-clinical administrative units, 15 are located in the School of Medicine, with the others distributed among three other Schools.

Researchers in basic science departments and ORUs do most of their research in "wet-lab" facilities, where they study animals, cells, and macromolecules: social science department researchers perform mostly "dry-lab" research, often involving computer analysis of patient outcomes vs. treatments or other variables, assessed from a variety of sources. The former bring in more research grant dollars (in total direct costs, TDC): $96 and $88M for basic science and ORUs, respectively, vs. $20M for social science. Research in wet-lab departments employs many more postdocs and occupies more research space than do dry-lab departments like Epidemiology and Biostatistics. The latter department, with many sponsored faculty, few postdocs, and relatively few square feet of research space, nonetheless garnered $12.6M in FY2014 research funds (see below).

Heterogeneities within unit subtypes are also striking. For ORUs, differences in faculty numbers (3-fold range) and sponsored research funds (10-fold) reflect their histories as well as the relative ability of particular research themes to attract funds. In Table 8-2, compare the Cardiovascular Research Institute (CVRI, which studies heart disease) or the Diabetes Center to the Institutes for Health and Aging, for Health Policy Studies, or the Proctor Foundation (for research in ophthalmology). Among ORUs, the CVRI has the most faculty and next to the top number of sponsored research dollars; UCSF's first ORU, it enjoys generous funding from an endowment dating back to the ouster of UCSF's Chancellor, engineered by the CVRI's leader in

Table 8-2. Basic Science Departments, Social Science Departments, and ORUs, FY2014

Dept/ORU*	Sch*	Spons Fac*§	Spons rsrc*§ (TDC)	Spons Rsrc* (IC)	Post-docs*¶	Space*‡ (asf)
		No.*	$M*	$M*	No.	Sq ft (K)‡
Basic Sci depts*‡‡						
Cell/Tissue Biol*	D	13	5.42	2.37	28	20.6
Anatomy	M	12	9.67	3.86	28	33.2
Biochem/Biophys*	M	15	19.1	6.67	71	92.6
CM Pharmacol*	M	12	12.8	5.21	55	42.0
Microbio/Immuno*	M	10	12.2	4.34	29	35.0
Physiology	M	9	6.57	2.20	40	38.4
Bioeng/Ther Sci*‡‡	P/M	25	13.9	9.55	60	48.3
Pharm Chem*	P	16	16.5	6.09	65	68.4
All		112	96.1	35.9	376	379
Social Sci depts*						
Anthro/Hist/Soc*	M	4	0.490	0.099	1	1.23
Epidemiol/Biostat*	M	53	12.6	2.85	11	17.3
Phys Nurs*	N	15	3.74	1.51	8	4.41
Soc/Behav*	N	13	3.25	0.766	—	3.70
All		85	20.4	5.22	20	26.6
ORUs						
CVRI*	M	19	21.6	8.48	60	108
Diabetes Center‡‡	M	11	38.7	8.93	39	18.9
HDFC Cancer C*	M	5	8.50	4.29	14	26.2
Health and Aging*	N	14	2.72	1.15	—	13.6
Health Policy*	M	12	5.47	1.42	2	12.8
Hooper Foundn*‡‡	M	—	—	—	4	7.58
Neurodegen Dis*	M	6	6.74	2.48	11	39.7
Proctor Foundn*	M	6	4.37	1.12	2	8.56
All		73	88.2	27.9	132	228
All units		270	205	69.1	528	633

Legend for Table 8-2 opposite page

the 1960s (chapter 7 and reference *13*). The Diabetes Center, with the highest number of research dollars and a middling number of sponsored UCSF faculty, attracts unusually generous funding from federal and non-federal sources for collaborative research projects that bring dollars to researchers at UCSF and other institutions. Also, several ORUs with lower research dollars are quite young. Similar differences in history and scope probably account for heterogeneity among social science departments.

Heterogeneities among basic science departments are less striking, but real. With the largest research space, postdocs, and sponsored research funds, Biochemistry and Biophysics was the first basic science department to focus primarily on research, when William Rutter became its chair in 1969 (*13*); it helped foster expansion and regeneration of research in other basic science

*Abbreviations: Anthro/Hist/Soc, Anthropology, History, and Social Medicine; asf, Assignable Square Footage; Basic Sci depts, Basic Science Departments; CVRI, Cardiovascular Research Institute; Cell/Tissue Biol, Cell and Tissue Biology; Biochem/Biophysics, Biochemistry and Biophysics; Bioeng/Ther Sci, Bioengineering and Therapeutic Sciences; CM Pharmacol, Cellular and Molecular Pharmacology; depts, departments; D, M, P, N, Schools of Dentistry, Medicine, Pharmacy and Nursing, respectively; Epidemiol/Biostat, Epidemiology and Biostatistics; HDFC Cancer C, Helen Diller Family Comprehensive Cancer Center; Foundn, Foundation; Health and Aging, Institute for Health and Aging; Health Policy, Philip R. Lee Institute for Health Policy Studies; IC, indirect costs; Lad rank, Ladder rank; Microbio/Immuno, Microbiology and Immunology; Neurodeg Dis, Institute for Neurodegenerative Disease; No., number; ORU, Organized Research Unit; PhD std, PhD students; Pharm Chem, Pharmaceutical Chemistry; Phys Nurs, Physiological Nursing; Postdocs, postdoctoral scholars; Sci, Science; Space, Research Space; Sch, School; Spons fac, Sponsored faculty; Spons rsrc, Sponsored Research; Soc/Behav, Social and Behavioral Sciences; $M, millions of dollars; TDC, total direct costs.

§Sponsored faculty are those who received any dollars from sponsored research projects in FY2014, as recorded and cited in chapter 6. For sponsored research dollars (Total Direct Costs, TDC) received by each unit's faculty, see reference 10.

¶The postdoc numbers were as of 1 January 2015 (11).

‡Research space is assessed by UCSF's analysts as assignable square feet (asf) used to support sponsored activity at the end of each fiscal year, and includes office space assigned to PIs with active sponsored activity in the fiscal year, as well as all rooms classified as laboratory research space (wet, dry, and support space). See reference 12.

‡‡Several apparent anomalies merit explanation, including (besides HHMI support, described in the main text): (i) the Diabetes Center's very large amount of sponsored research dollars, which reflects very large grants awarded to one of its faculty members; (ii) Bioengineering's faculty all belong to the School of Pharmacy, but the Department shares space from the Schools of Medicine and of Pharmacy, and part of its total sponsored TDC ($10.9M) is administered through the School of Medicine. (iii) The Hooper Foundation has space and postdocs, but its faculty are listed as members of other departments and their sponsored support is administered in those departments.

departments since the 1980s. Basic science department research is more vigorous than their sponsored research dollars indicate, owing to a happy anomaly, the Howard Hughes Medical Institutes (HHMI). In basic science departments, HHMI supports 14 faculty; they receive substantial sponsored funds from non-HMMI sources as well, but their departments' recorded sponsored funds include neither HHMI-paid salaries for faculty and some staff, nor HHMI-derived research funds (14). So, while UCSF basks in the HHMI's reflected radiance, departments with HHMI-supported faculty conduct more research than their sponsored dollars (Table 8-2) indicate. In FY2014, HHMI supported six faculty in Cellular and Molecular Pharmacology; three in Biochemistry and Biophysics, three in Physiology; and two in Microbiology and Immunology (15).

Table 8-3. Basic Science Faculty Salaries (PhDs only), FY2014: UCSF Compared to US Medical Schools*

	Assistant professors			Full professors		
	No.[‡]	Median salary $K[‡]	Ratios (UCSF/ Other)[#]	No.	Median salary $K	Ratios (UCSF/ Other)[#]
School(s)*						
UCSF[¶]	27	118		65	225	
All US[¶]	4061	92	1.29	4270	168	1.34
Public[¶]	2165	89	1.33	2165	161	1.40
Private[¶]	1896	98	1.20	1895	182	1.24

*Basic science department faculty (PhDs only) in UCSF's School of Medicine (UCSF) are compared with PhDs in the same type of department in US medical schools (All), and with those in schools funded by public (Pub, usually state) funds or by private funds (Priv). Data is from the AAMC (16). The AAMC data on basic science salaries includes neither faculty in the Schools of Dentistry, Pharmacy or Nursing, nor MD faculty with primary appointments in basic science departments.

¶Median values for total annual compensation are shown as thousands of dollars per year, and include total income (before taxes or set-asides for retirement) but not benefits paid by the University. While the AAMC records two classes of income, Fixed and Total, we show only the AAMC-defined Total income here, because in basic science departments, at UCSF and elsewhere, Fixed and Total values differ by an average of 1% or less. Fixed compensation is the amount fixed at the beginning of the year and contractually obligated to the faculty member. Total compensation includes, in addition to the fixed/contractual component, bonus or incentive pay that results from achievement of specific performance goals by the individual, the department, or the institution; examples may include bonuses from a faculty practice plan or outside earnings limited or controlled by the institution.

#Ratios are calculated by dividing UCSF's total compensation for assistant or full professors by the corresponding compensation for that rank in the AAMC category (all US, public, or private medical schools) shown.

‡Abbreviations: No., number of faculty assessed in a category; $K, thousands of dollars.

Faculty salaries

In principle, the dean of each School distributes salary money (from the state appropriation) and assigns space (offices, seminar rooms, and laboratory space, etc.) to each department or ORU. Within constraints imposed by available resources, chairs or directors of these units then distribute the dollars and space to individual faculty members in ways that differ in details among units, based on custom and need.

PhDs in basic science and ORU faculty PhDs at UCSF are well paid: salary comparisons for assistant or full professors show that UCSF pays this group 20-30% more than the average US medical school, public or private (Table 8-3; *16*). Because magnitudes of those differences persist in comparing the 75th percentiles of these groups (not shown), salaries of UCSF basic science faculty match those of counterparts in upper echelons of respected US research universities. Still, UCSF's basic science faculty salaries are constrained in critical ways:

1. In FY2014, faculty researchers in basic science departments and ORUs paid, respectively, 51 and 59% of their salaries from sponsored research projects (see Table 6-3, above). Their salaries are competitive, but legislators continue to shrink state funds for paying them. As competitors abound and NIH funding stagnates, PIs are distracted from real research by scribbling multiple grant requests in hope of receiving a single award, which may then be consumed to pay their own salaries.
2. San Francisco's high (and still climbing) housing costs make it extremely difficult to buy a small house on a basic science assistant professor's median UCSF salary ($118,000; Table 8-3; *16*), even combined with a spouse's salary (Box 8-1). Superb young scientists, unfortunately, can find acceptable jobs in less expensive cities.
3. House prices pose a subtler problem: senior professors bought houses 15-20 years ago, enriching them well out of proportion to the ~$108,000 salary difference between their median UCSF salaries and those of assistant professors (Table 8-3; *16*; and see below)—a disproportion, oppressive to the young but often invisible to their elders, that can generate resentment and stifle communication.

As in most academic biomedical research centers, at UCSF basic science departments determine the size of a faculty member's salary by beginning with the university's prescribed salary scale for each department, based on academic rank and responsibilities of specified groups of faculty. Every year the department chair and the individual faculty member negotiate a somewhat higher salary for that year (Box 8-2).

Basic science departments and ORUs find money to pay those negotiated salaries in complicated ways. They can pay salaries from three sources: (i) the state educational appropriation (SEA), supplemented by dollars from the Dean's office; (ii) sponsored research funds of the individual faculty member; (iii) department "reserves" (discretionary funds or endowments. For most basic science departments, the first two sources are critical, the third minuscule, though Biochemistry and Biophysics has a modest endowment and that of the

Box 8-1. Attracting and recruiting scientists

For half a century, UCSF found it easier than many rival institutions to attract the best and brightest young people. In the 1960s, it was still a fairly ordinary institution, but California's climate, scenery, and opportunities for adventure combined with state resources to attract doctors, scientists, and students from all over the US to the Parnassus campus (13). When UCSF began be seen as a potential leader in research, education, and patient care, it could compete successfully for recruits against richer and more illustrious institutions.

Now, however, UCSF's basic scientists express grave concern about the institution's continuing ability to attract bright young talent, from students and postdocs to faculty researchers. Graduate program directors say many top candidates choose competing schools, because prospective students who otherwise place UCSF at the top of their lists cannot afford to live in the Bay Area. UCSF offers them apartments at rents well below market rates, but available apartments are too few to meet current demand. In May 2015, rent for the average one-bedroom apartment ($38,600 per year, $3,213 per month; 17), exceeds the annual student stipend of $32,500 and is barely 10% less than the yearly salary of a first-year postdoc (18). Prospective basic science assistant professors (beginning salary, ~$110,000) quail at $1.0M+ mean house prices (mid-2015). Driven by rapid growth of Bay Area technology companies, the mean price rose 12% since 2012 and is predicted to rise a further 6% by mid-2016 (19).

Housing is a "very high priority for UCSF," according to Daniel Lowenstein, UCSF's Executive Vice Chancellor (20). Over the next 15 years, he adds, UCSF will focus on constructing, renovating, or purchasing apartments and offer them at rates much lower than the San Francisco market, primarily to students and postdocs. He expects UCSF will increase the present number of apartments at least three-fold; many will be located in or near the Mission Bay and Parnassus campuses, in renovated space owned by the university, or in purchased or newly constructed buildings.

Recruiting young faculty poses complex, longer-term problems for UCSF. "It isn't just finding a house, because young couples also seek assurance that they can find good schools for their children, all the way from pre-school day-care to college and beyond," says Joe Derisi, chair of Biochemistry and Biophysics (21).

Other basic science leaders worry that prospective basic science faculty members are not eager to assume the significant a long-term risk that depends on where the dollars come from—from the university vs. a less secure "soft" source, like NIH grants. Science professors in some universities may be surprised to hear that a basic science appointment does not obligate UCSF to pay more than ~50% of total salary. Most medical schools, however, do require rely basic science faculty researchers to provide substantial proportions of their salaries from grants. A survey (22) conducted for the Association of American Medical Colleges reported "extramural salary expectations" at nine top-ranked US medical schools. Although the schools were identified only by letters (A through I), we suspect that Harvard and UCSF were among them. Five of nine schools said they expected average basic science faculty to obtain 70-75% of their salaries from extramural sources, and one reported an expectation of 100% after three years on the faculty; the remaining three schools reported such average expectations of 25%, 40-60%, or 60%, respectively. Thus UCSF basic science faculty do earn high salaries, comparable to those paid in other top medical schools, as noted above, and their average soft-money support (~50%; chapter 6) is less than that expected at seven of nine (anonymous) medical schools. We do not have good data to compare UCSF's soft money for basic science salaries to "extramural salary expectations" of most universities for their PhD biologists or biochemists. It does appear likely that declining institutional support for academic salaries at UCSF and other medical schools adds yet another obstacle to recruiting and retaining faculty.

CVRI, an ORU, is quite substantial.

Now we turn to university-supplied SEA and Dean's office contributions, and proceed later to grants. From the 1970s until the early 1990s, the SEA supplied "Full Time Equivalent" (FTE) dollars, which paid ~75% of the average salary and benefits of basic science department professors in the ladder-rank series. (Most basic science faculty members were ladder-rank faculty, and still are; see chapter 6.) In the 1990s, diminishing SEAs gradually reduced the dollar value of FTEs, so departments had to ask faculty to tap their grants for larger proportions of salary—to 50% or even more, as compared to the earlier ~25%. In the 21st century, state funds dropped still further and grant money also became scarcer than before, leading to increasing financial deficits for departments, which (in the School of Medicine) were defrayed by separate yearly subventions from the Dean's office to each department.

To stabilize faculty and programs, basic science department chairs and the Dean of Medicine devised a new Basic Science Funding Model (BSFM), which first took effect in FY2015. Its key elements (25) include: (i) an executive committee (the Dean and basic science department chairs) reviews the

Box 8-2. Setting the salary of a UCSF basic science professor

Following UCSF's Faculty Health Sciences Compensation Plan, salaries in departments and ORUs are determined in three stages:

1. *X factor.* The university prescribes minimum salaries for full-time faculty, depending on academic rank and a salary scale (Scale 0 to Scale 9), assigned by departments to individual faculty according to their academic responsibilities, recognizing that "departments with limited revenue will not have enough money to fund a high covered [compensation] . . . supported by departmental income and taxes" (*23*). Most faculty in basic science departments or ORUs are compensated on Scale 3. Rank and scale determine the "X" component of each faculty member's salary.

2. *Y factor.* Each year the department chair negotiates with the individual faculty member to set the "Y" salary component. Y is a multiplier that brings the individual's salary from the X value to a value (X+Y) that meets the negotiated target (see main text), which is that year's contracted salary, constrained by available funds.

3. *Z factor.* This salary component is a bonus or incentive that conforms to university rules and available funds. For faculty discussed in this chapter, most Z dollars are compensation for consultation for an external company or institution; few basic science faculty members earn appreciable Z compensation, so the Z component contributes on average less than 1% of total earnings.

Most university-paid benefits (e.g., UC retirement and health care insurance) are fixed as a percentage of the X component of a faculty member's salary.

(Note: This account omits many details; for a less streamlined account, readers may subject themselves to the rigors of UC's Academic Personnel Manual; *24*.)

model at regular intervals and advises the Dean on allocation of vacant faculty slots; (ii) rather than having to depend solely on FTEs of diminishing value and ad hoc Dean's office subventions, each department gets an annual block allocation from the Dean's office, including a base administrative allocation ($335,000 per year, identical for each department) plus ladder rank allocations for each position, depending on ranks of individual faculty; (iii) allocations for

Table 8-4. Basic Science Funding Model
vs. Faculty Salary Needs

	Model	Equiv* endow- ment[§]	Actual salary (avg*)[¶]	Salary+ benefits (avg)[‡]	Model rel to actual*[#]
	$K*	$M*	$K	$K	%
Faculty salaries					
Assistant Professor	75	1.5	118	153	49
Associate Professor	85	1.7	145	188	45
Full Professor (1-5)[§§]	105	2.1	225[§§]	292	36
Full Professor (6-A)[§§]	130	2.6	225[§§]	292	45
Administrative salary[##]	50	1.0	92.5	120	38

§Assuming payouts of 5% per year, these are the values of endowment principal that would be required to pay the model salary amount.

¶Actual faculty salary is based on AAMC records (16) of UCSF's median salaries for these three ranks in FY2014.

‡Salary + benefits calculated by multiplying the actual salary by 1.297.

#The proportion paid by the model allocation is calculated by dividing the model's allocation by the actual median salary for that rank or position.

‡‡Actual administrative salary is calculated as described in reference 32, assuming an average of 29.7% for benefits.

§§Full professors are paid on scales with incremental steps, increasing from 1 to 5 and finally (at the top) above scale (A). The table compares each of these only with the average actual salary (at all possible scales) for full professors at UCSF.

*Abbreviations: Avg, average; equiv, equivalent; $K, thousands of dollars; $M, millions of dollars; rel to, relative to.

faculty positions include separate components for their salaries and administrative support (Table 8-4); (iv) block allocations are to the departments, not to individual faculty; (v) vacant FTEs revert to the Dean's office, with their associated funds distributed through the block allocation to the departments; (vi) chairs reach a consensus to recommend recruiting into vacated positions. Codicils (26) largely follow custom and precedents of earlier years. The Model provides, depending on rank, between 36% and 49% of actual median salaries paid to UCSF basic science faculty in FY 2014 (Table 8-4); the remaining 51-64% must come from grants.

A federal "salary cap" could limit use of grant dollars to pay salaries of highly remunerated basic science professors at UCSF (and of a much higher proportion of clinical department faculty, as shown in the next chapter). This federal salary cap—the maximum salary federal grants can pay any individual grantee—was lowered in 2011 from $199,700 to $179,700, and rose slightly in 2014, to $181,500. The 2014 cap would not pose a serious threat to the

Box 8-3. Running a basic science department on the BSFM

To ask how a basic science department can or cannot function on the new Model, we compare expenses and "income" of a fictional UCSF basic science department, with 12 ladder-rank faculty members: two assistant professors, two associate professors, and eight full professors. The department's total expenses, $2,442,500 per year, include:

- Faculty salary plus benefits, based on average salaries for these ranks in basic science departments, come to a total of $3,000,000 (28). If (as estimated in reference 25) the BSFM were to cover 48% of assistant and associate professor salaries and 41% of professor salaries, the BSFM would pay $1,280,000 for department faculty salaries, while sponsored projects would pay $1,720,000 (29).
- Mandatory charges from UCSF Human Resources, pro-rated to the department's number and type of employees: $125,000 per year (30).
- Mandatory charge for pre-award administration of grant applications, pro-rated for type of application: $300,000 (30).
- Mandatory charge to support graduate programs, $4,250 per student x 30 students in departmental laboratories: $127,500 (31).
- Miscellaneous unavoidable charges (32): $130,000
- Administrative salaries for four personnel, x $120,000 (including salary and benefits) for each (33): $480,000.

Another expense is the basic science departments' contribution to support of adjunct faculty who plan, coordinate, and teach courses for medical students. Amounts of these contributions are substantial and vary greatly among the different departments. Such adjunct faculty have been supported in part by Dean's Office subventions, but some basic science departments lack resources necessary to pay the rest of the tab.

Income. The BSFM would supply a total of $2,195,000 per year, including $1,260,000 to support faculty salaries, plus $600,000 for their staff, plus a departmental "base" of $335,000 (34).

Inevitable deficit. With the expenditures above, the department must end the year $247,500 in arrears (= $2,442,500 - $2,195,000)—a deficit higher than "reserves" available to the department. Reserves, in theory, include endowments and grant dollars awarded for faculty salaries, if they exceed what the university agrees to supply via the BSFM. To pay that $247,500 deficit from endowment, at an annual 5%payout rate, the endowment principal would have to be $4.95M—much more than the endowments of most basic science departments. The department could require its faculty to provide the $247,500 by increasing the overall percentage of their salary supplied from grants by an additional 14%, from $1,720,000 to $1,967,500. A final alternative: the department could dismiss two of its four administrative personnel, saving ~$240,000 per year. No alternative is attractive.

In devising the BSFM, the Dean's office and department chairs clearly under-estimated the costs of faculty salaries and staff salaries and mandatory or unavoidable administrative costs. Actual faculty salaries of the fictional department, including benefits, amount to $3,000,000, for which the BSFM explicitly provides $1,260,000, or 42% overall. As its executive committee planned from the outset, the BSFM will have to be re-adjusted. Probably the Dean's office will supply extra funds to help pay inescapable administrative costs and staff salaries; sponsored projects may also have to pay somewhat larger proportions of faculty salaries higher than guessed earlier.

average UCSF basic science professor, who in FY2014 earned $225,000 per year (16; and Tables 8-3 and 8-4): with benefits equal to 29.7% of total salary, she would need a total of $292,000, of which $105,000 could come from the BSFM. To collect the remaining $187,000 of the $292,000 from federal grants, her grants would have to support $144,000 in actual salary plus $43,000 in benefits (29.7% of $144,000). That $144,000 is 64% of her $225,000 salary, but also ~21% less than the current NIH salary cap. What if she and her basic science department chair were instead to negotiate a very high salary— i.e., the maximum in BSFM dollars ($130,000; Table 8-4) plus the maximum allowed by the salary cap? Combining both sources, such a professor would earn a maximum of $281,500 in actual salary (27). Of 112 sponsored faculty in UCSF's basic science departments in FY2014, at least nine (8%) received gross salaries higher than $281,500 in 2014 (27).

The BSFM was devised to stabilize faculty salaries, but has so far not done so. This is because its dollars conspicuously do not suffice for departments to pay unavoidable charges incurred by carrying out their research and teaching and also maintain a minimal staff (see Box 8-3); as a result, some departments have to "tax" faculty salary dollars supplied by the BSFM to support essential departmental functions.

Table 8-5. Basic Science Departments: Faculty, Space, Sponsored Dollars, and Ratios*‡§

	Fac	Space¶	Spons $		Per faculty: Spons $	Space	Per space: Spons $	
		asf	TDC	IC	TDC+IC/ Fac	asf/ Fac	TDC/ asf	IC/ asf
	(No.)	(K)	($M)	($M)	($K)	(No.)	($)	($)
Cell/Tissue Biol	13	20.6	5.42	2.37	417	1585	263	115
Anatomy	12	33.2	9.67	3.86	806	2767	291	116
Biochem/Biophys	15	92.6	19.1	6.67	1271	6173	206	72
CM Pharmacol	12	42.0	12.8	5.21	1063	3500	304	124
Microbio/Immunol	10	35.0	12.2	4.34	1222	3500	349	124
Physiology	9	38.4	6.57	2.20	730	4267	171	57
Bioeng/Ther Sci	25	48.3	13.9	5.26	556	1932	288	109
Pharm Chem	16	68.4	16.5	6.09	1031	4275	241	89
All	112	379	96.1	40.0	858	3379	254	95

*Abbreviations: Exactly as in Table 8-2, plus the following: Fac, Faculty; Spons, Sponsored; K, thousands; $K, thousands of dollars; $M, millions of dollars; No., number

§Sponsored faculty, sponsored research dollars, and space are defined as described in the legend of Table 8-2, which also describes where the information was obtained.

‡Notable anomalies include those described in the legend to Table 8-2. It should be noted that the fortunate anomaly of HHMI support, described in the main text, misleadingly reduces the sponsored dollars and thus reduces the dollars per faculty member and the sponsored dollars per asf for departments that have HHMI faculty. The Hooper Foundation is omitted from this table sponsored support of its faculty is administered by other departments.

¶For definitions of research space and Assignable Square Footage (asf) used by UCSF's analysts in this table and elsewhere in this chapter, see Table 8-2 legend and reference 12.

Research space

Next to research dollars and salary, academic researchers tend to worry most intensely about adequate (that is, bigger) space for their laboratories. Consequently, research institutions seek dollars to construct and maintain research facilities, with an intensity matching their devotion to recruiting first-rate scientists. Different subtypes of non-clinical academic units—basic (Table 8-5) and social science (Table 8-6) departments, and ORUs (Table 8-7)—deploy researchers and research space in distinctive ways. Taken together, "basic" departments (narrow definition) have the most sponsored faculty members, research space, and sponsored research dollars: 112 sponsored faculty vs. 85 for social science, and 73 for ORUs; 379,000 assignable square feet (asf) vs. 228,000 for ORUs, and much less (~27,000) for social science; $132M in re-

Table 8-6. Social Science Departments: Faculty, Space, Sponsored Dollars, and Ratios*§

	Fac	Space	Spons $		Per faculty: Spons $ Space		Per space: Spons $	
		asf	TDC	IC	TDC+IC/ Fac	asf/ Fac	TDC/ asf	IC/ asf
	(No.)	(K)	($M)	($M)	($K)	(No.)	($)	($)
Anthro/Hist/Soc	4	1.23	.491	.099	147	308	399	80
Epidemiol/Biostat	53	17.3	12.9	2.85	298	326	749	165
Phys Nurs	15	4.41	3.74	1.51	349	294	847	341
Soc/Behav	13	3.70	3.24	.767	308	285	876	207
All	85	26.6	20.4	5.22	302	313	767	196

*Abbreviations are as described in the legends of Tables 8-2 and 8-5.
§Sponsored faculty, sponsored research dollars, and space are defined as described in the legend of Table 8-2, which also describes where the information was obtained.

search TDC + IC vs. $116M for ORUs and ~$26M for social science departments.

Within each category, heterogeneities abound (Tables 8-5, 8-6, and 8-7). Among basic science departments, Biochemistry and Biophysics (School of Medicine) has much more asf and somewhat more sponsored dollars than its near competitors in the School of Pharmacy (Bioengineering and Therapeutic Sciences and Pharmaceutical Chemistry), one of which has more sponsored faculty. Among social science departments, Epidemiology and Biostatistics has by far the most faculty members and sponsored dollars. Among ORUs, the CVRI has 2.5- to 11-fold more space than other ORUs and also more sponsored funds, with one exception, the Diabetes Center (owing to grants awarded to one of its faculty; see Table 8-2 legend).

Comparing the three types of non-clinical academic units to one another offers more useful lessons, specifically with respect to ratios of sponsored research dollars to asf or faculty numbers (Fig. 8-1). First, social science departments (including Epidemiology and Biostatistics) have about as many faculty as do the other two unit types, but very much fewer asf, making their collective asf-faculty ratio less than one seventh the mean for non-clinical departments at UCSF (Fig. 8-1, top left panel). Sponsored dollars per social science faculty member are also lower, but the difference is less marked than the asf difference: relative to means for all non-clinical departments, means for social sciences are 30% or 24%, depending on whether TDC or IC is compared (Fig. 8-1, two right upper panels). Most strikingly, social science departments gar-

Table 8-7. Organized Research Units: Faculty, Space, Sponsored Dollars, and Ratios*§

	Fac	Space	Spons $		Per faculty: Spons $	Space	Per space: Spons $	
			TDC	IC	TDC+IC/ Fac	asf/ Fac	TDC/ asf	IC/ asf
		asf						
	(No.)	(K)	($M)	($M)	($K)	(No.)	($)	($)
CVRI	19	108	21.7	8.48	1587	5684	201	79
Diabetes Center	11	18.9	38.7	8.93	4332	1718	2049	472
HDFC Cancer C	5	26.2	8.50	4.29	2558	5240	325	164
Health & Aging	14	13.6	2.72	1.15	276	971	200	84
Health Policy	12	12.8	5.47	1.42	574	1067	428	111
Neurodeg Dis	6	39.7	6.74	2.48	1436	6617	170	62
Proctor Foundn	6	8.56	4.37	1.12	916	1427	511	131
All	73	228	88.2	27.9	1590	3120	387	122

*Abbreviations are as described in the legends of Tables 8-2 and 8-5.
§Sponsored faculty, sponsored research dollars, and space are defined as described in the legend of Table 8-2, which also describes where the information was obtained.

ner 2- to 3-fold greater sponsored research dollars per asf than basic science departments. This difference reflects different ways of conducting research: as compared to basic science, social science departments (i) focus on dry-lab rather than wet-lab research; (ii) use sponsored faculty to carry out higher proportions of actual research, so that (iii) smaller groups (and many fewer postdocs; Table 8-2) tackle each problem; (iv) expect individual sponsored faculty to attract smaller amounts of sponsored dollars, so that (iv) one asf of (predominantly) dry-lab research space brings the university three times more TDC dollars and double the IC dollars earned in one asf of predominantly wet-lab space. The comparisons also suggest that wet-lab research leads to greater recovery of indirect costs (per TDC dollar) than does dry-lab research, which may reflect greater reliance on private funding for the latter. Further, we speculate—the necessary data are not yet available—that, paradoxically, research in dry-lab space may actually incur less indirect cost for the institution to pay (per TDC dollar), because dry-lab research uses smaller teams of scientists and less space and technical equipment.

How do ORUs fit into this comparison? Their apparent ability to bring in almost twice as many sponsored TDC dollars per asf (on average) than basic science departments (Fig. 8-1, lower panels) may partly reflect dry-lab research approaches (e.g., in Institutes for Health and Aging and for Health Policy), but not in intensively wet-lab ORUs like the CVRI. Again, more careful analysis is in order.

Note that a substantial and increasing, but not yet quantitated, proportion

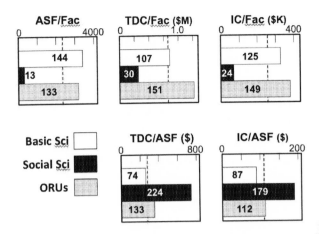

Fig. 8-1. Space and research dollars in Basic Science and Social Science departments and in ORUs, in relation to number of faculty and to each other, FY2014.

Top panels show research space (in asf, or Assignable Square Footage) and sponsored dollars (total direct or indirect costs—i.e., TDC or IC) per the numbers of sponsored faculty members (Fac) in each type of administrative unit (see chapter 6 and Tables 8-2 and 8-5 to 8-7). Bottom panels show TDC or IC per research asf for these same units. Numbers within each bar show the relation of the absolute value in that bar (as a percentage) to the mean value for all three classes of unit together; these mean values are depicted as vertical dashed lines in each panel. Abbreviations are as in the legend of Table 8-2.

of research in UCSF's clinical departments applies dry-lab approaches, and thus requires more sponsored faculty (and probably fewer postdocs) per sponsored dollar. It will behoove UCSF's leaders to pay attention to these changes (see chapter 9). Note also (and again) that quantitative comparisons—e.g., sponsored ICR dollars per asf—are not always valid. For instance, in FY2014 three of eight basic science departments brought in less than the $90/asf specified in the UCSF policy described in chapter 4, and only two would meet the $120/asf requirement for 2016 (Table 8-5). Such arbitrary cut-offs could result in ignoring anomalies like HHMI funding and can tempt leaders and researchers to pay less attention to a more critical concern: quality of the research itself.

Research training

After obtaining her bachelor's degree, an aspiring biomedical scientist begins learning to do science as a PhD student and then as a postdoctoral scholar. Both stages focus on performing laboratory research directed by an academic scientist, and together can last 10-12 years, or even more. PhD aspirants

Table 8-8. Estimated Research and Training Costs in Non-clinical Departments*

Faculty		
Number[§]		270
Salaries[¶]		
Sponsored	$M	24.4
Intramural	$M	22.6
Total	$M	47
Sponsored research[§]		
TDC	$M	216
IC, recovered	$M	69
(IC, unrecovered)	$M	34
Total		319
Training		
Graduate students (basic sciences)		
Number[‡]		670
Student costs[‡]	$M	33
Postdocs (~500+)		
Number		~508
Salaries[‡]	$M	~24

*The data provides a general overview of all non-clinical departments at UCSF. The data are not related precisely to one another, in that some refer to FY2014 and others to 2013 or 2015, as noted below. The categories also overlap, in that the total dollars for sponsored research include (but are not limited to) dollars that paid faculty salaries, supported PhD training, or paid postdocs.

§Faculty number and sponsored dollars include basic science and social science departments plus ORUs, based on data in Tables 8-5, 6, and 7, above.

¶Faculty salaries are taken from chapter 6, Table 6-3.

‡Data for graduate student numbers refer to FY2013 (35). Postdoctoral salaries are estimated by multiplying the number of postdocs at UCSF (in 2015; 11) by the salary NIH stipulated for third year postdocs in FY2014; 18, 44). The cumulative cost of UCSF's student tuition, fees, and living stipend is based on estimates of $33M for basic science PhD students, as described in the main text.

can easily opt for more lucrative careers with shorter preparation times, so biomedical PhD programs routinely pay their students' tuition and fees, plus stipends of $30,000-40,000 for living expenses. Postdoctoral scholars pay no tuition or fees and receive bigger (but still niggardly) stipends, set by NIH at ~$42-55,000 per year, depending on experience (18).

Producing young scientists is expensive. In UCSF's non-clinical departments, it costs about $33M per year to train a PhD pipeline of ~670 basic science PhD students, and ~$24M to pay about 500 laboratory postdocs (Table 8-8). The ~$57M devoted to both stages of training exceeds the total combined salaries of sponsored faculty in those departments, and comes to 18% of total (estimated) sponsored research costs in laboratories of basic science departments and ORUs. (Caution: in comparing such costs, note that research and training costs partially overlap; see Table 8-8 legend and text below.) The training dollars produce good scientists. Career outcomes of UCSF's PhD alumni are more successful than the national average: 78% obtain research jobs in academia, industry, or government, with only 3% in non-scientific occupations, as compared to national figures, respectively, of 69% and 13% (*36*). UCSF's postdoctoral alumni probably also fare well; the percentage of alumni engaged in actual research is likely to exceed the 67% national average in 2012 (*37*). Now we turn to our focus on funding, and touch on salient issues regarding both stages of training.

Training PhD students. In 2013 UCSF trained 670 PhD students (*35*) in ten separate basic science training programs (*38*) and 165 in five social science training programs in 2014, including 94 students in the Nursing PhD program (*39*). In 2015, the annual average cost per student for basic science programs is ~$50,000, including tuition and fees of ~$16,800 and (for basic science students) a $32,500 stipend for living expenses (*40*); total cost would thus come to ~$33M per year (~670 students times $50,000); average time-to-degree is 5.92 years (*41*). The annual cost for training social science PhDs is not available but is certainly lower, because student numbers are smaller and social science PhD programs may not all support their students at rates comparable to those of basic science programs. Graduate programs in both categories differ considerably in size and time-to-degree. Among basic science programs, times-to-degree vary from ~5.2 to ~6.2 years (*41*).

Where does this money come from? Here we could obtain only very rough estimates (*42*): the ~$33M annual cost for basic science programs appears to be paid from three sources: (i) roughly 30% from UCSF itself, principally from the Chancellor's office to the Graduate Division, plus smaller amounts from UCSF's four Schools; (ii) roughly 40% is paid by extramural sources, including individual student fellowships and institutional (federal) training grants; (iii) finally, roughly 30% is paid from research project grants (RPGs) to support students working in labs of UCSF PIs. Overall, of 2015's estimated $33M total cost, these percentage estimates suggest these sources provide, very roughly, $10M from the institution, $10 M from fellowships and training grants, and $13M from extramural sources.

Because the estimated 30% from RPGs goes exclusively to students in later years of PhD training, a shorter average time-to-degree would disproportionately diminish the drain on PIs' research funds. If so, why do UCSF's

PIs persist in paying approximately $10M of their RPG dollars for graduate student stipends? The most likely answer: UCSF's PhD students in their later training years not only provide skilled labor, but also constitute a workforce as creative and strongly motivated as any a PI is likely to find elsewhere, and at a relatively cheap price. Moreover, that price is dictated by market competition: most other major biomedical research centers in the US pay living stipends similar to those paid at UCSF, plus tuition and fees that are often higher. Still, biomedical PhD students pay yet another price: that is, the length of graduate training may delay their careers as much as two years longer than is absolutely necessary, and that training may not always provide optimal learning opportunities for the brightest students (43). Thus market competition maintains the costs research centers pay to attract graduate students, and the need for cheap but highly motivated laboratory workers probably prolongs the years required to get a PhD degree. Chapter 10 will return to these issues.

In sum, for the past 25 years graduate training at UCSF has met with remarkable success. UCSF has raised the number and quality of its graduate programs, slowly reduced the time-to-degree (by perhaps more than half a year), and replaced many lectures in the first year with pedagogically effective workshop courses focused on specific problems and new research tools. It has also achieved the most critical goal, by training students who enjoy excellent career outcomes (36).

Postdoctoral scholars. As noted above, UCSF's basic science departments and ORUs paid an estimated $24M to 508 postdocs in FY2014 (see figure legend, Table 8-8, and 44). Still, labs in basic science and ORUs (in all UCSF Schools) employ in 2015 14% fewer postdocs than in 2005 (508 now vs. 592 earlier). For basic science and ORU labs in the School of Medicine, the decrease over that period was 18% (11)—paralleling decreases in inflation-corrected sponsored dollars over the same period: 10% for basic science departments in the School of Medicine, 16% for ORUs (see Fig. 7-1). San Francisco living costs that dismay prospective students and assistant professors may make it even harder to recruit postdocs to basic science labs.

Before we proceed to weightier matters, ponder this contrast: as an institution, UCSF appears to deem graduate students infinitely more valuable than postdocs, in that it pays approximately $10M from intramural funds for PhD students, vs. close to zero for postdocs, who receive (almost) all their salary from extramural grants. In part, this difference reflects UCSF's dedication to its educational mission. In contrast, however, PIs appear to assign almost identical economic values, in dollars per worker, to an average later-year graduate student and an average postdoc (44).

What is the future of basic science at UCSF?

Surveying their present predicament, faculty, students, and postdocs worry about the future. Exciting questions and technology offer limitless opportunity, but dicey dollars and insecure employment foster passivity and sap resolution. Of the four main causes for worry—three economic, one psychological—each increases the others' power.

1. Inflation and stagnant federal support make it hard for faculty to maintain their research momentum, and frantic scrambles for grant dollars weaken their appetites for tough but critical scientific questions.
2. Decreasing state appropriations for academic salaries may convert NIH's decision not to fund a grant request into loss of a research program or a PI's sudden inability to feed her family, and make it harder for departments to recruit students, postdocs, and new faculty—especially in competition with rich institutions or UC campuses with many undergraduates and thus higher state salary appropriations (Box 8-1).
3. Rapidly rising costs of housing and living in the Bay area lead prospective students, postdocs, staff, and faculty to seek—and often find—opportunities elsewhere.
4. UCSF's basic science community remains eager to share scientific goals and technology, welcome new ideas, and nurture young colleagues, but lacks its once keen interest in shared visions for the future and initiatives for constructive change.

How can we explain the current psychological malaise of UCSF's basic scientists? Pressed by tighter economic constraints, do investigators simply prefer the short-term solace of laboratory research to the thorny dilemmas of their communal future? As clinical medicine's prosperity grows, do deans and chancellors—like the society around them—pay less attention to scientists' triumphs or troubles? Do scientists suffer mainly from loss of their former autonomy and high regard? To what degree does their present insecurity reflect their much-diminished responsibility for teaching professional students? Do pride and self-pity promote exaggeration of troubles less dire than at other institutions? Are basic scientists spoiled aristocrats who should pull up their socks at once, and devise new ways to adapt and prosper?

Each harsh interpretation contains a tiny kernel of truth, but none offer cogent explanations of the present predicament or straightforward remedies.

As with most real-world problems, variables are many, causes hard to prove, and actions replete with risk. After chapter 9 examines research in clinical departments, chapter 10 will suggest approaches for dealing with some predicaments, but not all.

Chapter 9

Science in clinical departments:
Ambition vaults to success

The size, variety, and sponsored funding of research in UCSF's clinical departments make analysis difficult. By every measure, the clinical departments' research dwarfs that of basic science departments: 6.3-fold more sponsored clinical research faculty; 4.6-fold more sponsored funding; 2.3-fold more research space; 4.0-fold greater proportional growth over the past 11 years (1). A major contributor to the success of clinical department research at UCSF is the rapid expansion and growth over the past three decades in size, dollars, and social-political power of the entire US clinical enterprise and—in direct parallel, and even more successfully in financial terms—of UCSF's clinical enterprise (see chapter 1). This expansion: (i) attracted many clinician-researchers—both unfledged and well established—who competed effectively for research support and recognition against researchers in other institutions; (ii) drove an increase in professional fee dollars, earned by the clinical prowess of clinicians, which provided modest funds essential for boosting progress of research projects less strongly supported (after 2004) by federal dollars; (iii) helped persuade both NIH and private funders to target greater proportions of their portfolios toward clinical and translational research.

Clinical department research is impressive in quality as well as quantity. In the 1970s through the 1990s, UCSF's clinical departments made major advances in pioneering surgery for tiny fetuses in the mother's uterus, preventing cardiac arrhythmias by ablating cells in small areas of the human heart, inventing the clinical hospitalist (now a key contributor to patient care in many large centers), and discovering tobacco company cover-ups of smoking's dangers (which provoked medically critical changes in public policy). This quality and diversity persists in the 21st-century (see examples in Table 9-1; 2). Several advances reflect careful analysis of pathogenesis, especially of disorders of immune responses and the brain. Some are "basic," others clearly "applied,"

**Table 9-1. Research in UCSF Clinical Departments:
21st Century Examples***

1. Gene expression tests identify pathogenic mechanisms in asthmatic patients, point to specific therapy (John Fahy and Prescott Woodruff; 3)
2. Identification of genes causing episodic neurologic disorders, including sleep, altered circadian rhythm (Louis Ptacek, Ying-Hui Fu; 4)
3. Dissection of immunologic mechanisms in multiple sclerosis, leading to more specific and effective therapy (Stephen Hauser; 5)
4. Identification of genes that control development of neurons and other brain cells and their roles in brain injury (David Rowitch; 6)
5. The role of a type of lymphocyte, the ILC2 cell, in triggering allergic responses to many stimuli (Richard Locksley; 7)
6. Advances on multiple fronts in treating and preventing AIDS (spearheaded by Robert Grant, Diane Havlir, and many others; 8)
7. Acting as a prion, α-synuclein causes Multiple System Atrophy, a neurodegenerative disease (Stanley Prusiner; 9)

*These examples were culled from suggestions by 18 leaders and researchers at UCSF. Because most of these individuals claimed knowledge only of advances in their own fields (2), the authors suspect that at least one non-overlapping table could present advances comparable in number and quality to those listed.

but all aim to benefit patients, in the near term or later.

Of the advances in Table 9-1, only the AIDS-focused example reflected research primarily oriented to patients or involving dry-lab analysis (e.g., epidemiology, clinical management questions, etc.). The table probably does not reflect the true quality (or abundance) of UCSF's patient-focused research, for a curious and critical reason: the 18 individuals in clinical departments asked to recommend advances for this table (including department chairs, division chiefs, and even first-rate scientists in clinical departments) proved almost universally unable to cite recent discoveries or advances outside their own field or clinical unit; this reticence was even stronger among dry-lab researchers (2). Interviewees deemed deserving candidates for the table too numerous for any clinical department scientist to know. In sharp contrast, almost every faculty member interviewed in the smaller, better-integrated basic science community readily expressed a judgment (see Table 8-1). The difference points straight to sheer size of the clinical enterprise, which directly reflects the diligence and ability of its faculty, but appears also to hinder their opportunities, and perhaps even their motivations, for exploring science outside their immediate purviews. We shall return to this issue.

The rest of this chapter considers three aspects of clinical department research: (i) how administrative units manage the flow and distribution of

Table 9-2. School of Medicine, FY2014: Patterns of Research Funding, by Department Type*

Funders	Federal		Private clinical trials		Private C&G		Private total (trials + C&G)		Federal + Private	
	TDC+ IC $M**	IC¶ $M (%)	TDC+ IC $M	IC $M (%)	TDC+ IC $M	IC $M (%)	TDC+ IC $M	IC $M (%)	TDC+ IC $M	IC $M (%)
Dollars										
Clinical	389	78.6 (20)	25.5	5.28 (21)	149	23.0 (16)	174	28.3 (16)	563	107 (19)
Basic	81.5	22.3 (27)	0.404	0.068 (17)	17.0	2.87 (17)	17.4	2.94 (17)	98.9	25.2 (26)
ORU	83.1	21.5 (26)	0.993	0.163 (16)	22.6	3.95 (21)	23.6	4.11 (17)	107	25.6 (24)
All UCSF	553	122 (22)	26.9	5.51 (20)	188	29.9 (16)	215	30 (16)	769	158 (21)
Proportion within dept type (%)#										
Clinical	69		4.5		26		31		100	
Basic	82		0.41		17		17		100	
ORU	78		0.92		21		22		100	
All SOM	72		3.5		24		28		100	
Proportion of Federal + Private sponsored total (%)§										
Clinical	50		3.3		19,4		22.6		73	
Basic	10.6		—		2.2		2.2		13	
ORU	10.8		0.1		2.9		3.1		14	
All SOM	72		3.5		24		28		100	

*FY2014 sponsored funds in the categories listed are tabulated in reference 10. Unlike tables in chapters 7 and 8, this data includes only departments or ORUs that are located within the UCSF School of Medicine. These include seven basic science departments and five ORUs, plus 20 clinical departments and other units (in categories defined by the UCSF Chancellor's office; see 11). The data includes only funds derived from federal donors (principally NIH) or private funds (e.g., foundations or industry); funds from the state or local government are not included. In addition to regular clinical departments, the "clinical" category includes 7 School of Medicine administrative units designated as "other" in Figs. 7-2 and 7-3. These other units include the AID Research Institute, the Center for Health and Community, the Clinical and Translational Sciences Institute (CTSI), the office of the Medical School Dean, Human Genetics, the Osher Center, and Regeneration Medicine; altogether, these units account for 5.1% of the School of Medicine's sponsored funds, of which the CTSI accounts for nearly two thirds. The table does not separate these from regular clinical departments for two reasons: (i) to simplify the discussion, based on the low proportion of sponsored funds in the School of Medicine these units receive; (ii), like clinical departments, the "other" units are oriented towards research on a disease or a discrete set of clinical problems, and are geographically close to UCSF's clinical facilities on the Parnassus campus.

¶IC (indirect costs) are given in millions of dollars and as a percentage (in parentheses) of the sum of total direct costs plus indirect costs.

#These proportions represent total + indirect costs under a particular funding heading (federal, private clinical trials, private C&G, or total private funding, or all federal + private funds), as a percentage of the total sponsored funds received by the indicated department type (basic, ORU, clinical, or "all SOM").

§These proportions represent total + indirect costs under a particular funding heading (federal, private clinical trials, private C&G, or total private funding, or all federal + private funds), as a percentage of the total sponsored funds (federal + private) received all SOM administrative units; that total amount in FY2014 was $769M.

**Abbreviations: C&G, contracts and grants; TDC, total direct costs; IC, indirect costs; $M, millions of dollars; ORU, Organized research Unit; SOM, School of Medicine.

research dollars to scientists; (ii) competing research styles (dry-lab vs. wet-lab, clinical vs. basic science); (iii) training clinician researchers. Finally, we summarize our findings and identify challenges clinician researchers now face.

Where the dollars flow

We begin by asking how faculty and administrators obtain grant and contract dollars from external sources, how internal funds are channeled to separate administrative units and individual researchers, and how faculty salaries are paid.

Dollars from external sources. Table 9-2 documents the predominant role of research in clinical departments in UCSF's School of Medicine. As earlier chapters indicated, at UCSF three of every four sponsored dollars (73%, in FY2014) support research in clinical departments. In dollar terms, clinical departments garner greater than 5-fold more sponsored funds than do basic science departments or ORUs. For private (non-federal) funds, the difference is even greater: $174M to clinical departments, vs. $17M to basic science and ~$24M to ORUs (10- and 8-fold greater, respectively). This difference is not due to clinical trials: while basic science departments and ORUs participate in few clinical trials, privately sponsored clinical trials account for less than 5% of sponsored funds going to clinical departments (*10*). Clinical departments also participate in federally-sponsored clinical trials (not shown as a separate category in Table 9-2), but such trials pay UCSF only ~$15M per year, making up ~4% of the $389M per year (TDC+IC) clinical departments get from federal funders (*10*). Clinical departments recover proportionately fewer indirect cost dollars than other department types (Table 9-2), because clinical departments derive more of their sponsored funds (31% vs. 17% or 22% for basic science or ORUs) from non-federal sources, which reimburse indirect costs at lower rates (see chapter 3).

Researchers in clinical departments depend on federal grants for 69% of their sponsored funds (Table 9-2). Such funds come in many grant types (*12*), including several frequently used in basic science departments, such as RO1 grants for specific research projects, and PO1 or "project grants" in which multiple labs approach complementary aspects of a larger scientific problem. More familiar to clinician researchers, sometimes almost exclusively so, are federal grants designed especially for large projects aimed at understanding and treating clinical problems, including: P30 Center Core grants, P50 Specialized Center grants; clinical trials, which usually involve more than one institution; and U-grants (cooperative agreements in a specified area of research, which often fund large projects involving multiple institutions). U-grants often result from requests for applications aimed at a programmatic objective of an NIH center or institute, but may also originate from curiosity or interests of individual researchers or groups of researchers in a particular field. Most NIH K-awards for training go to clinician scientists, although some go to researchers in basic science departments.

In mid-2013, a high UCSF official told one of the authors that the days of curiosity-driven research were numbered. Instead, the official said, the old model was being rapidly replaced by institutional "resource aggregators" (a group to which he proudly belonged) who work in concert with industrial funders to organize university investigators, basic and clinical, into consortiums focused on large research projects. Although UCSF had already hosted many projects funded by private industry, such projects did increase in number and size with following the appointment of Susan Desmond-Hellmann, an outstanding clinical investigator from Genentech who served as UCSF's Chancellor from 2009 to 2014 (13). UCSF is now engaged in research agreements with multiple industrial partners, which include Pfizer, Genentech, GE Healthcare, Nikon Instruments, Abbott Diagnostics (14), and others. Private (non-governmental) funds also come to UCSF from drug company-sponsored clinical trials (see above), and a host of foundations and philanthropists. The "research aggregator" probably exaggerated, although we were not able to estimate accurately how many dollars industrial partnerships contributed to UCSF's privately sponsored funds in FY2014 (Table 9-2).

What makes clinical departments so much better at attracting research funds than other UCSF department types? The causes are not amenable to quantitation or experimental tests (see Muddlement Uncertainty Principle in chapter 6), including:

1. The expanding clinical enterprise provides many recruits who are active researchers.
2. Clinical departments have access to professional fees, which pay substantial parts of their salaries and may also be used, in limited amounts, to support research. As federal dollars shrank, these "extra" dollars became much more valuable.
3. Clinical departments can truthfully point to their daily work and expertise as reasons for philanthropy aimed at near-term improvements in human health and welfare.
4. Responding to voters, Congress and NIH target federal dollars to clinically relevant "translational" research based on hopes that short-

term efforts can quickly transform untapped reservoirs of basic knowledge into cures for disease.

5. UCSF's clinician-researchers eagerly take advantage of new federal initiatives, such as NIH requests for applications, Clinical and Translational Sciences Institutes, support for clinical research centers, and large "cooperative agreements" (U-grants).

6. Past partitioning of academic clinical medicine into specialty silos (e.g., cardiology, neurology, rheumatology, etc.) created compartments in which small groups of highly motivated clinician-researchers can mobilize resources and personnel to tackle targeted goals, through: (i) multi-center collaborative trials involving many patients and subsets of clinical specialties; (ii) dry-lab approaches to understanding and treating disease; (iii) K-awards and other grants to convert MD-PhDs, young resident physicians, and specialty fellows into investigators who perform research in UCSF labs and clinics and go on to research positions at UCSF and elsewhere.

For various reasons, all these advantages have proved inaccessible and/or less attractive to PhDs in basic science departments (see chapters 7, 8 and 10).

Administering research in the medical school and its departments and divisions. The School of Medicine accounts for ~85% of all expenditures of UCSF's campus (*15*) and is also responsible for most of both its clinical income and its research. From the Chancellor, its Dean's Office gets a modest portion of indirect costs on sponsored projects and distributes these directly to departments in proportion to the ICR each generates. Although the Dean has little or no direct clinical income, his office plays major roles in supporting research and teaching throughout the School. Fig. 9-1 diagrams six discrete sources of that office's revenues and shows how that money was distributed among three uses: operations of the Dean's Office itself, medical education, and—most important—support of programs (*16*). Most of the $31M devoted to program support was derived from the Dean's Tax and interest and investment income ($25M and $17M, respectively; a dotted box in Fig. 9-1 surrounds those two sources). Although professional fees of different departments are taxed at somewhat different rates (see Fig. 9-1 legend), on average this tax in FY2014 came to 5.6% of the $449M of such fees, which are collected by the clinical enterprise and distributed to departments in proportion to their faculties' clinical earnings (*17*).

In FY2014 almost all program support went either to clinical departments ($13M, which included $6M in packages for recruiting department chairs and

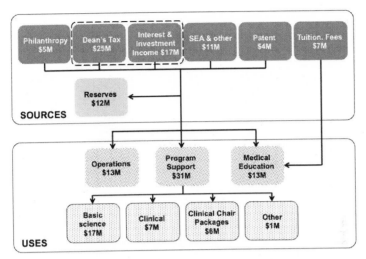

Fig. 9-1. Sources of Dean's Office funds and their use for operating and program support in the UCSF School of Medicine, in FY2014 (16). Boxes (in the top row, and the third and fourth rows) represent, respectively: sources of Dean's Office dollars; large categories of uses, including operations of the office, medical education, and support of specific school programs; and four categories of program support. The "Reserves" box ($12M, in the row just below the top row) represents dollars held in reserve (and earning interest) for use in future years. The dashed line around the Dean's Tax and Interest and Investment Income boxes indicates the sources of most program support. Of this program support, $13M was used for clinical department programs and to prepare packages for recruiting chairs of clinical departments. The basic science department category includes dollars for specific basic science department programs, some funds for graduate education, and supplementation of arrears in department budgets for that year. [In FY2015, an amount similar to the last of these items will be combined with some State Educational Appropriation (SEA) funds to support the Basic Science Funding Model, described in chapter 8.] The Dean's tax itself ($25M) represents the average 5.6% "tax" on professional fees of $449M (17); in reality, different individual clinical departments are subjected to Dean's taxes of different percentages, based on decades-old agreements between Deans of Medicine and those same departments.

$7M of other purposes, including research and new programs) or to basic science departments ($17M). Of these, the $17M for basic science is devoted to recruiting new and retaining current faculty, support of selected research endeavors, some funds for PhD education, and making up arrears in the accounts of six of the seven basic departments (18), which lack the necessary reserves and endowment income to pay all their faculty and administrative personnel (see chapter 8). In FY 2015, the annual "arrears" of basic science departments will be defrayed by the Basic Science Funding Model (see chapter 8), using dollars drawn from sources similar to those in Figure 9-1.

Dean's Office support for programs in basic science departments represents a bone of contention for many clinical leaders and faculty. A senior clinical department faculty member told one of the authors that many clinical colleagues fear that "the basic sciences are bleeding us white"—a fear based, apparently, on four perceptions: (i) the $17M is greater than the sum received by highly regarded, fiscally prosperous, and much more populous clinical departments; (ii) the $17M is derived mostly from clinical professional fees, with no contribution from basic science faculty; (iii) UCSF clinicians' salaries lag behind those of their counterparts in other universities, while UCSF basic scientists earn more, on average, than most academic basic scientists (Table 8-3, above, and see below); (iv) assignable square footage of prime research space occupied by basic science laboratories on the Mission Bay campus is disproportionately greater than that devoted to clinical research (measured in relation to numbers of research faculty, to sponsored research funds, or to indirect cost dollars (19). (For research space, see chapters 7 and 8, Table 7-4, and Fig. 8-1; its distribution has not yet been analyzed with respect to use for dry-lab vs. wet-lab approaches.)

Although we began by discussing dollars from the Dean's Office, the Dean of Medicine does not directly control research in clinical departments. Instead, "the departments, along with their divisions, determine the numbers of their research faculty, depending on space and departmental income," says a knowledgeable senior department chair (20). The Dean appoints department chairs and may influence how much research space they control, but department chairs and division chiefs make all key decisions related to hiring, paying, evaluating, and retaining faculty. In this respect, US medical schools differ, he says. "In some other schools, the dean must approve all faculty hires. But at UCSF, research-intensive clinical departments, and often their divisions, function as distinct entities which may collaborate with one another but in many ways operate as separate silos." Research-intensive departments include Medicine, Pediatrics, Pathology, and Neurology. Within departments, certain divisions (often bigger than small departments) are especially research-intensive (21).

Several clinical department chairs say their departments comprise "two separate economies." In the larger economy, focused on patient care, faculty receive guaranteed salaries plus incentive supplements that depend on extra clinical activity, and participate modestly in research. In the research economy, faculty spend ~30% of their time in clinical work, following the dictum that an active research program requires a 70+% time commitment; most (but not all) their remaining income is derived from research grants. Each economy is said to be governed by a wryly termed "eat what you kill" principle, where "kill" denotes salary incentives for clinical productivity or grant dollars that sustain the bulk of a researcher's salary. (We shall return to salaries in a moment.)

In practical terms, clinical departments and divisions derive their incomes from multiple sources. One source is professional fees earned by their faculty members, which are taxed not only by the Dean but often also by departments and sometimes by divisions; some units need pay no more than 90% of their professional fees as faculty salaries, and so can devote the rest to other purposes, while poorer units may devote virtually all professional fees to faculty salaries. Units are "rich" or "poor," depending on: (i) the actual amount of their professional fees (among specialties, incomes differ markedly); (ii) ability to attract philanthropy (i.e., endowments from patients or their families may pay part of the salary of an individual faculty member, be devoted to a designated purpose, or serve as general support at the discretion of a unit's director); (iii) ability to attract sponsored research funds from private, state, local, and federal sources, including the small proportion of indirect costs that trickles down to individual administrative units; and (iv) quite limited support from the state. Each unit uses dollars from these various sources to support multiple activities, including—in addition to research—unit administration, supplementing faculty salaries; improving patient care; teaching students, residents, and fellows; recruiting new faculty; and supplementing pay of trainee researchers (see K-awards and research training, below). With so many variables at play, it is not surprising that research is stronger and better supported in some departments and divisions than in others.

Similarly, it should not surprise that researchers in clinical departments disagree about the quality of their research environment and its administrative support. In response to our request to nominate projects and scientists for listing in Table 9-1, one clinician-researcher noted (22) that "big scientific discoveries don't seem to be high on clinical department chairs' radar screens," and added, in a later interview, that "UCSF should squeeze the hospital harder than it does" to support research and other academic missions. In broad agreement, another clinician-researcher (23) felt that the Teaching Hospital's leadership must "buy in to research as an important function, not just as an occasional tool for implementing new ways to save money." But "this they don't do—at least, not yet," owing to "the big gap between the medical school and the hospital." Others take a more sanguine view, pointing to widespread success of clinical department research and its ability to attract bright young people and make them into highly productive scientists. One leader argues that the "silo problem" has a potentially brighter face: compartmentation into

Table 9-3. Clinical Department Faculty Salaries (MDs only), FY2014: UCSF Compared to US Medical Schools*

| | Assistant Professor | | | Full Professor | | |
	No.[‡]	Median salary $K[‡]	Ratio (UCSF/ Other)[#]	No.[‡]	Median salary $K[‡]	Ratios (UCSF/ Other)[#]
"Fixed" salary[¶]						
UCSF[¶]	490	175		442	255	
All US[¶]	34,456	178	0.98	14,326	244	1.05
Public[¶]	17,072	167	1.05	7,875	231	1.10
Private[¶]	17,384	190	0.92	6,451	255	1.00
"Total" salary[¶]						
UCSF[¶]	490	189		442	266	
All US[¶]	35,033	228	0.83	14,401	298	0.89
Public[¶]	17,632	220	0.86	7,947	288	0.93
Private[¶]	17,401	235	0.80	6,454	312	0.85

*Clinical department faculty (MDs only) in UCSF's School of Medicine (UCSF) are compared with MD faculty in clinical departments of US medical schools (All), or with those in schools funded by public (Pub) funds or by private funds. Data from the AAMC (27). The AAMC data on clinical department faculty salaries includes neither faculty in the Schools of Dentistry, Pharmacy or Nursing, nor PhD faculty with primary appointments in basic science departments.

¶Median values for total annual compensation are shown as thousands of dollars per year, and include total income (before taxes or set-asides for retirement) but not benefits paid by the University. The AAMC records two classes of income, Fixed and Total: fixed compensation is the amount fixed at the beginning of the year and contractually obligated to the faculty member; total compensation includes, in addition to the fixed/contractual component, bonus or incentive pay that results from achievement of specific performance goals by the individual, the department, or the institution; examples may include bonuses from faculty practice plan or outside earnings limited or controlled by the institution. We show both classes of income data here because in clinical departments they differ substantially, as the table shows. (In a previous chapter, the comparable table—i.e., Table 8-3—for PhD basic science faculty showed only the AAMC-defined total income, because in basic science departments the values differed by an average of 1% or less, at UCSF and elsewhere.)

#Ratios are calculated by dividing UCSF's fixed or total compensation for assistant or full professors by the corresponding fixed or total compensation for that rank in the AAMC category (all US, public, or private medical schools) shown.

‡Abbreviations: No., number of faculty assessed in a category; $K, thousands of dollars; UCSF, University of California, San Francisco; US, United States.

separate clinical specialties allows investigators to probe in original and innovative directions, which can prove highly productive (24).

Faculty salaries. One reason clinical departments have trouble recruiting young researchers from other institutions, according to two chairs of research-intensive clinical departments (25, 26) is that UCSF doesn't pay salaries high enough for young clinicians to live in the ultra-expensive Bay Area. This problem, they agreed, also limits recruitment and retention of clinical stars. Indeed, median UCSF clinician salaries are lower than median salaries at medical schools in places where living costs are lower, as shown for MD assistant and full professors in UCSF's clinical departments in FY2014, vis-à-vis those in other US medical schools, public and private (Table 9-3; 27). At both ranks, so-called median "fixed" salaries—i.e., those guaranteed for the coming year—are similar at UCSF to those at public and private medical schools. But fixed salaries in medical school clinical departments are significantly lower than "total" salaries, which include incentive dollars earned by clinical productivity. By the "total" measure—most relevant for a person considering a new job in a particular city—assistant and full MD professors in UCSF's clinical departments earn median salaries lower (by 7-20%, depending on the comparison; Table 9-3) than their counterparts in other US medical schools. (Table 9-3 does not compare salaries for physicians in specific subspecialties.)

Underlying causes for these differences in total salary are not clear. Does UCSF need to raise incentive supplements to clinical salaries? Or do San Francisco's attractions, over time, induce an excess of clinicians to look for jobs in the area, allowing the local market to hire aspirants at lower salaries than elsewhere? If so, UCSF may have attracted young physicians at those lower salaries more easily in previous years, before living costs rose so rapidly (see chapter 7). Also, it is worth noting that UCSF faculty must somehow find ways to live in the same city, whether they are MDs in clinical or PhDs in basic science departments. For the former, median total assistant professor salaries in FY 2014 were 60% higher than median salaries of assistant professors in basic science departments; for full professors, the difference (18%) was lower but still substantial (compare Tables 9-3 and 8-3).

Clinical department researchers in the in residence series, which does not guarantee a university salary, earn much of their salary from sponsored projects. One senior physician scientist, Kevin Shannon (28), sees proportionately large "soft-money" salaries as drivers of "a virtuous cycle." His division of pediatric hematology/oncology has 17 faculty members whose salaries are 60% supported (on average) from research grants. "As a result, we have 17 faculty to share a clinical job that might require seven, if they saw patients every hour of their work-day. That means we have extra time to pay careful attention to the sickest patients and to teach students and residents—a real win/win!" [Often expressing the opposite view, UCSF's basic science researchers fondly recall an era (20 years ago) when they needed to earn only ~25% of their salary from grants, and the state took care of the rest; see chapter 8.]

Clinician researchers and their chairs now confront a different threat, from the $181,500 federal salary cap—i.e., the maximum salary, set by Congress, that federal grants can pay any grantee (see chapter 8). It does not materially affect academic clinicians, who can earn whatever the clinical enterprise charges for their services. But clinician-researchers (and others) strongly believe that a satisfactory research program requires 70% of a faculty researcher's time. If so, for a clinician researcher who gets 30% of her salary for clinical work and the rest from grants, maximum "take-home" salary would be $181,500 ÷ 0.70, or $259,571 per year—a number slightly greater than the $255,000 median "fixed" salary received by UCSF's MD full professors, and ~$6,500 less than the $266,000 median "total" (that is, incentivized) salary of MD full professors.

The dilemma is straightforward: without a subsidy, one of every two professor-rank faculty researchers in UCSF's clinical departments receives more than the median full professor salary, and so cannot maintain her/his income from clinical earnings and grants alone. Half of all full professors (and a greater fraction in low-earning clinical specialties) are unaffected by the NIH salary cap, but the other half must scramble to find that subsidy, and scramble harder if they belong to a highly paid specialty. For now departments pay necessary subsidies from reserves, professional fees, endowments, and other philanthropy. But it is not hard to imagine a further arbitrary reduction in the federal cap (increased to its present level in early 2014, by barely $1,000; see chapter 8), and increases in median salaries are surely inevitable. In either case, like most other medical schools, UCSF will face a troubling quandary: should the institution reduce take-home salaries of many clinical researchers, require them to derive more than 30% of salary from the clinic, or subsidize their salaries with money diverted from different purposes? None of these approaches is attractive.

Wet- vs. dry-labs: how shall these twain meet?

Profound economic and organizational changes in US medical care drive a revolution that is slowly transforming UCSF's three central missions: not only patient care and medical education, but also research. Explicitly recognizing that revolution, UCSF's new "Bridges Curriculum" for medical education (slated for implementation in 2016) will augment traditional "foundational sciences" (which gave their names to basic science departments, including Epidemiology) with "emerging sciences (e.g., clinical informatics, change management, continuous quality improvement, metacognition, public and global health, systems engineering)" that are crucial for patient care in complex health care systems and for improving health of populations (29). These changes in patient care also drive the growth and immense complexity of the UCSF clinical enterprise, with profound effects on research. In clinical departments, prominent effects are expansion and growing strength of patient-oriented "dry-lab" research. Here we compare and contrast wet- and dry-lab research and explore consequences of the latter's growth.

Wet-lab research. Until about 1990, almost all research in UCSF's clinical departments focused on understanding the biology of disease. In departments like medicine, pathology, pediatrics, and neurology, researchers eagerly jumped on the DNA bandwagon, with gratifying success in studying and developing therapies for certain kinds of disease; other kinds, of course, proved harder to crack (*30*).

Moreover, as we might expect, individual silos created by clinical departments and their divisions may be better suited for tackling some problems than for others. In general, for instance, a particular silo may lack broad interactions with disparate experts needed to explore mysterious pathogenic mechanisms, like those underlying psychiatric disease or inflammatory bowel disorders. But the same silo, or a different one, may offer precisely the right focus and collaborative intensity required to explore therapeutic approaches, under either of two special circumstances, when: (i) an anatomical site or a new technology provides unique opportunities for diagnostic or therapeutic advances—e.g., in electrophysiology of arrhythmias, microsurgery, or radiologic diagnosis and guided interventions; (ii) disease pathogenesis is better understood and more amenable to truly translational research, as in some types of cancer, infectious diseases, or immune disorders (*30*). In this respect, rheumatology and infectious disease divisions in UCSF's Department of Medicine are unusually strong. Not surprisingly, these two divisions have also actively explored and contributed to collaborations with faculty in basic science departments; in other cases, collaborations are comparatively rare.

Clinical departments and divisions have trouble fostering wet-lab research for two more reasons. First, most of UCSF's wet-lab clinician-researchers are home-grown, not recruited from other institutions, because (*26*): (i) the national "market" for wet-lab clinicians is weak, owing both to a dearth of excellent scientists and to their tendency to remain where they were trained, as they do at UCSF; (ii) recent increases in San Francisco's cost of living make it even harder to hire young scientists; (iii) clinical departments choose not to risk the substantial expenditures (start-up costs, salary, laboratory space) required to recruit a young scientist before her/his long-term success appears assured. This third possible cause is discussed further below.

Dry-lab research. As mentioned earlier, so-called dry-lab (or patient-focused) research in medical schools refers to many different kinds of goals and projects, all focused on disease and patients. These may include epidemiology of disease or injury in relation to environmental or other variables (e.g., smoking and lung cancer); clinical tests (from measurements of uric acid or electrolytes to genome analysis) as markers of diseases or their outcomes; implementation of new management standards or therapies; clinical trials; costs vs. benefits (e.g., in dollars, distress, deaths vs. longevity, patient satisfaction, level of function) of diagnostic or therapeutic approaches.

Patient-focused research has strong roots at UCSF, dating back to the late 1970s (*31*). It received a large financial and organizational boost in 2006, with a large NIH grant ($109M over five years) to found UCSF's Clinical and Translational Sciences Institute (CTSI); by 2016 the renewed grant (2011) will have brought $112M to UCSF. Mike McCune, the CTSI's first director, explains that clinical research requires more collaboration and longer delays between posing initial questions and getting good answers, and, because it focuses on humans, is based on less detailed biological knowledge and cannot perform certain kinds of experiments. So, UCSF's CTSI sought initially to establish training and infrastructure and build a coherent clinical and translational research community at UCSF within 15 years (*32*). Now a large part of CTSI's grant (*33*) supports courses and other training of young clinician researchers and promotes independent creative activity by awarding small grants to young scientists to initiate promising projects. A third goal was to promote increased productive research interactions between researchers in clinical and basic science departments.

Of these goals, expansion of training has met the most success. To be fair, the Department of Epidemiology and Biostatistics was already teaching courses in methods and practice of "dry-lab" research, but these were expanded and now extend to more students. Offerings include summer workshops and formal courses in statistics and epidemiology, an internship in translational research, mentoring of individual clinical research projects, a master's degree program, a doctoral program, and programs for clinical K-awardees (*34*). Former students in many of these courses rate them highly; now, as clinician faculty members at UCSF, many use what they learned in successful research (see K-awards and training, below). The small-grant program has also made a positive impact by helping young clinical researchers. Efforts to bring basic science and clinical department researchers together gained little traction, owing to lack of interest on the part of some basic scientists, geographical separation of the two groups on different campuses, and the irreplaceable roles of actual conversation and mutual potential advantage in initiating productive collaboration—roles websites and internet connections can never play as effectively.

The financial or space "footprints" of dry-lab research in clinical departments at UCSF are substantial and have almost surely expanded over the past decade. Jeffrey Olgin, chief of the division of cardiology (Department of Medicine), estimates that 50% of the division's faculty researchers employ predominantly "dry" approaches in their research; of incoming cardiology fellows, he says, 70% prefer "dry" to more biological (wet-lab) approaches (24). To our knowledge, however, no one has yet quantitated dry-lab vs. wet-lab science in any UCSF context.

Nonetheless, as compared to wet-lab research, dry-lab research should appeal to space- and dollar-strapped chairs and division chiefs for two reasons: smaller start-up costs; personnel costs and square feet of research space are also smaller at the outset of individual projects, although they grow if the research succeeds. Medical students and many resident physicians, clinical fellows, and would-be clinician researchers may also prefer the goals and methods of dry-lab research, because it: (i) has greater relevance to sick patients; (ii) is more in keeping with their previous training; (iii) in short time frames, is more likely to succeed; and finally, (iv) requires shorter training than the MD-PhD route followed by most wet-lab researchers, thus imposing shorter delay (by 4-5 years) before research independence is achieved (see training, below).

Neither CTSI's efforts nor dry-lab clinical research receive high marks from all clinical faculty, however. Three clinical aficionados and successful practitioners of wet-lab clinical science all levy some version of at least two of the following criticisms: (i) bright young K-awardees may profit from CTSI courses, but the courses cost their divisions or departments too much money; (ii) the CTSI has not effectively improved UCSF faculty access to sources of "big data," whether in terms of genomes, specific mutations, clinical profiles, or any other information (one investigator opined that in this regard UCSF is far behind leading biomedical research centers); (iii) CTSI teaches techniques for assessing data, but does not try to teach students to distinguish between useful/interesting questions and dull questions of the "me-too" variety. (Dry-labbers expressed no opinions, and near-zero interest, with regard to wet-lab research.)

It is hard for non-experts (like the authors) to judge whether wet-labbers' criticisms are correct, but it seems possible that wet and dry camps are pitching their tents on opposite sides of a ravine that can divide them for some time. Such a ravine recalls a disturbing parallel gulf between basic and clinical department researchers.

Table 9-4. K-awards in the Department of Medicine, 2003-2012*‡

Issue	Data		
155 total K-awards received¶	32% were at Parnassus; 28% at San Francisco General Hospital; 40% in other DOM units, including ORUs		
Where they were in 2013	124 at UCSF (120 still in DOM) 30 (~20% of total) had left UCSF, including: 19 associate professors; 3 assistant professors; 3 private practice; 5 insufficient information		
K-award type§	58 K23 (mentored patient-oriented) 58 K01 (mentored research sci.) or K08 (mentored clinical sci.) 4 miscellaneous (1 K02, 2 K07, and 1 K22)		
Research funds, 2013§	Research funded for 99 at UCSF, including 50 with NIH grants		
Faculty series at UCSF, 2013#	Award begins: 2003-07	2007-10	2010-12
In residence	15	11	11
Clin-X or HSC	12	12	7
Adjunct	13	17	24
Total	40	40	42

*The table includes K-awards received by individuals in UCSF's Department of Medicine from 2003 to 2012. Its data was derived from a survey conducted in 2012-13 and reported to faculty and leaders of the Department in 2014 (40).

¶This number includes the 124 awardees still at UCSF in 2013, plus 30 who left UCSF. In the interim, one of the 155 awardees died.

§These include only the 120 awardees who remained in the Department of Medicine in 2013.

‡Abbreviations: Clin-X, Professor of Clinical X faculty series; DOM, Department of Medicine; HSC, Health Science Clinical faculty series; ORUs, Organized Research Units.

#The total number for whom faculty series was listed (122) is between the 120 still in the Department of Medicine as of 2013, and the 124 still at UCSF in the same year. We cannot determine the source of this apparent discrepancy, but it is too small to affect materially tentative inferences from the series data (see main text).

Training new scientists in clinical departments

Once upon a time, young science-inclined MD easily straddled the border between clinical medicine and biomedical science. But now it takes longer to acquire both sets of complex knowledge and skills, as well as credentials necessary to certify them. After college, a young person may devote 18 years to preparing for a combined clinician-scientist career in academia, at age 40 or even older. The once porous border has become a series of hurdles (Fig. 9-2, top bar): MD and PhD degrees, residency training, a specialty fellowship, and an uneasy period of candidacy for full faculty status, signaled by receipt of a five-year NIH K-award, also known as a "career development award."

Despite these exacting demands, hurdles persist, partly because many young people still take up the challenge: in the US, about 500 enter MD/PhD training every year, including, in 2015, 13 at UCSF (*36*). According to a 2010 survey of MD-PhD training at 24 US medical schools (*37*), about 90% of matriculated students finish MD-PhD training; of the graduates, 81% remain in academia, where most engage in research; on average, ~16% opt for private medical practice.

Medical schools have not effectively reduced the temporal burden on MD-PhD students, in part because making either a competent academic physician or a competent scientist is not easy. Judging clinical competence is straightforward, but it remains fiendishly hard to predict whether a budding scientist will succeed, and long-term investments in clinician-scientists are expensive. So, the university uses NIH K-awards to help decide whether or not to accept candidate clinician-scientists as full faculty members. According to the chair of one clinical department (*26*), the K-award period provides a period during which the NIH—first by awarding the K-grant and later by awarding (or not awarding) an RO1 research project grant—promotes or blocks a candidate's success. "By ourselves we can't judge quality or predict success well enough," he added, so faculty candidates are judged by this "Darwinian" selection—even though departments know NIH's judgments can be arbitrary and incorrect.

K-awards defray only part of the large cost of multi-year auditions of candidates for faculty status. At the outset, clinical department awardees are usually adjunct assistant professors receiving ~$130,000 per year, of which the K-award itself covers ~$80,000 (~60%); once awardees transfer into the in residence series, which signals faculty status, divisions usually contribute more, bringing total annual salary up to $150,000 and sometimes higher, depending on specialty (*38*). UCSF's clinical departments find that K-awards satisfactorily reduce the dollar investment they make. Indeed, they may pay (collectively) as much as $2M per year (= ~40 new K-awardees x $50,000) to first-year K-awardees, over and above the K-award. From 2006 to 2013, UCSF's scientists received 350 K-awards—40% more than the closest rival school (*39*).

In general, MD-PhD students are thought to become wet-lab investigators, although a recent survey shows that a small but increasing proportion conducts more patient-focused research (*37*). In any case, the (mostly) wet-lab scientist training track has a formidable rival in clinical departments at UCSF:

Table 9-5. CTSI Trainees in the K award program*

Responders*	63 total; 44 women, 19 men
Advanced degree(s)	45 MDs (includes 33 with other degrees also: 4 PhD, 29 MS or MAS); 12 PhD only; 5 other[¶§]
Institution type	58 in academia; 1 in industry; 1 in private practice; 3 other[#]

Entered program (year):	2005-07	2008-09	2010-11	Overall
No. in cohort[¶]	26	25	12	63
Position[‡]				
Assistant Prof[¶]	6 (23)	12 (48)	8 (67)	26 (41)
Assoc Prof[¶]	13 (50)	12 (48)	4 (33)	29 (46)
Prof[¶]	4 (15)	0	0	4 (6.3)
Non-academic/other	3 (4)	1 (4)	0	4 (6.3)
Effort (%) in C/T research[‡¶]				
0-20%	3 (12)	1 (4)	1 (8.3)	5 (8)
20-59%	9 (35)	6 (24)	0	15 (24)
≥ 60%	14 (54)	18 (72)	11 (92)	43 (68)
Research grants or contracts[‡]				
Any as Principal Investigator	24 (92)	21 (84)	12 (100)	57 (90)
NIH R03 or R21	2 (7.7)	5 (20)	0	7 (11)
NIH RO1 or equivalent	25 (96)	12 (48)	1 (8.3)	38 (60)
Industry	8 (31)	14 (56)	7 (58)	29 (46)
Foundation	9 (35)	3 (12)	0	12 (19)

Median no. of publications per respondent[¶¶]	
All publications	13
As first or last author	8

* Between October 2013 and December 2014, CTSI surveyed all individuals who had entered its K Scholars program between 2005 and 2011 and had completed their K award before the time of the survey (41). The 63 responders represent ~95% of the individuals who fitted these two criteria.

¶Abbreviations: Assoc, Associate; CTSI, Clinical and Translational Science Institute; C/T, clinical and translational; MAS, Master of Advanced Studies; MS, Master of Science; No., number; Prof, Professor.

§The five other degrees include: one Doctor of Dental Science; one PharmD, Doctor of Pharmacy; three ScD or DSc, Doctor of Science.

#Non-academic biomedical research institutions constitute the "other" category.

‡Data in all these categories (Position, Effort (%) in C/T research, and Research grants or contracts) was correct at the time of the survey. In each, the data shows the number of individuals and, in parentheses, their percentage within the cohort. Not surprisingly, awardees who entered the program earlier are more likely to have been promoted to the rank of Professor and to have received more research support from the NIH and industry. Conversely, % effort devoted directly to C/T research tends to be somewhat reduced for awardees who entered the program early, perhaps because older individuals gradually assume additional responsibilities, while individuals just out of training enjoy greater freedom to engage in research.

¶¶The number of publications refers to the median number published by all respondents; these are not divided with respect to cohort (year of entry into program). The order of authors on a scientific publication often indicates whether an author wrote the paper and performed the experiments (first author) or is the Principal Investigator who supervised and directed the research (often last author): authors listed between first and last author contributed to the paper but were (usually) not primarily responsible for it.

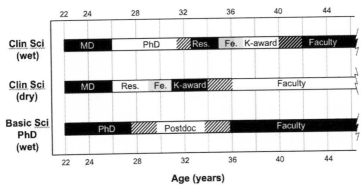

Fig. 9-2. Estimated duration of three alternative routes to becoming an academic biomedical researcher. These potential routes, from top to bottom of the diagram, include: in the top bar, Clinical Science, wet-lab [Clin Sci (wet)]; in the middle bar, Clinical Science, dry-lab [Clin Sci (dry)]; in the bottom bar, Basic Science, wet-lab [Basic Sci PhD (wet)]. Different stages in the transition from college graduate (at age 22; far left in the diagram) to faculty investigator (far right) include: four years for the MD degree; between 5.8 and 7.2 for the PhD degree; two to three years for medical residency (Res.); two years for specialty fellowship, which may include one year of research training (Fe.); K-award; postdoctoral scholar (Postdoc, five to eight years). Time estimates for these stages are not based upon objective data, but rather upon conversations with researchers. It should be noted that the variation in length of several stages is quite large—in some cases even larger than indicated than indicated by dotted or cross-hatched regions between certain stages in the diagram. More specifically: MD degrees usually take four years, but may be faster in MD-PhD programs; K-awards are usually for five years, but frequently overlap with faculty status at some point; residency training may require from two to five years; specialty fellowships from 1-3 years; probably the most variable durations are those required for PhD degree (6.5 years, on average, in the US; 35) and postdoctoral training (four to seven years, or even more).

to skip the PhD hurdle altogether, MDs can instead opt for dry-lab research, by joining the CTSI K-Scholar Program. This program teaches them dry-lab concepts and methods in courses on statistics, clinical trials, epidemiology, and health-care delivery and mentors each trainee's efforts to develop research programs in her own specialty. During the entire training period, trainee salaries are partially supported by individual K-awards or by an NIH K12 award, administered by the CTSI, and supplemented by the trainees' departments or divisions. This shorter track allows trainees to become full-fledged faculty and begin independent research by age 35 or 36, about the age PhD scientists begin independent research in basic science departments (compare middle and lower training tracks in Fig. 9-2, which presents rough time estimates; as noted in the legend, wide variations are not rare).

Overall, UCSF invests substantial energy and dollars to recruit young people in its residency and specialty fellowship programs into applying for

Table 9-6. Interviews with Recent UCSF K-awardees

Awardee	First UCSF position	Age at interview	Post-grad[¶] degrees	K-award (latest)	Wet vs. Dry Lab	Faculty rank	Research support
A	Med student	Early 40s	MS, MPH, MD	K23	Dry	Assoc prof (In res.)	RO1, K, & others

After residency and training in palliative care elsewhere, A took an adjunct assistant professor position at UCSF. Mentors and colleagues helped A to apply successfully for federal and other research funds, all focused on the geriatric patients A treats. In addition, A regularly blogs and tweets on how to improve care for these patients.

B	Faculty	Late 30s	MD, PhD	K08	Both	Assoc prof (In res.)	K08, RO1, others

To avoid the adjunct/K-award route (a sort of "purgatory"), at age 35 B moved to a UCSF faculty position from fellowship training in New York. Supported by a successful RO1 application, B's lab aims to improve treatment of a lethal disease. Advisers encourage B's strong lab commitment; clinical care contributions remain modest.

C	Residency training	Late 30s	MD, PhD	K12	Wet	Asst adjunct prof (In res.)	K12; appl. for K08

As a postdoc, C studies neural changes in a devastating brain disease. Now toiling to write papers and apply for a K08 award, C expects soon to look for a combined research and clinical position outside UCSF. Putting maximum energy into this effort, C worries the game may turn out to be "a pyramid scheme, after all."

D	Residency training	Early 40s	MD, PhD	K08	Wet	Asst prof (In res.)	K08, appl. for RO1

With strong departmental support, excellent research mentors, a strong publication record, and a small lab, D is working to secure federal funding and wishes the broader scientific community was more interactive. Working hard every day, D finds opportunities to discuss science are primarily confined to encounters with immediate colleagues or those with similar research interests. "Being an assistant professor at UCSF can be very isolating."

E	Specialty fellowship	Early 40s	MD	K08	Both	Asst prof (In res.)	RO1

Despite productive research, success in garnering federal grant support, and commitment to understanding and treating disease, E feels intellectually isolated and unsupported in a faculty enclave ("not real researchers; they mostly do what some company tells them") who don't need grants, owing to salary support from endowments. The school and department, E fears, do not appreciate how important research really is.

F	Specialty fellowship	Mid 30s	MD	K23	Dry	Asst prof (In res.)	K23

F found CTSI-taught courses useful, although often long-winded, and feels isolated from "dry-lab" scientists in other departments. Asked to identify highlights of dry-lab research at UCSF or nationally, F offered vague comments but little specific information. F finds patient-oriented research hard when health-care providers are reluctant to participate. Already a recipient of non-federal research funding, she now faces the challenge of channeling her pilot studies into fundable projects, including award of an RO1 grant.

G	Specialty fellowship	Early 40s	MD, PhD	K08	Wet	Asst prof In residence	K08

G's specialty fellowship at UCSF was coupled with research in a basic science department. Despite generous startup funds and a supportive division, G feels uneasy mixing wet-lab research with clinical work next to busy, very capable clinicians whose clinical earnings contribute to G's salary. Chairs and division chiefs tell G they rely on NIH peer review to judge young scientists' work, which they cannot do themselves, but G feels it should be "their job to take on some of the risk, decide for themselves, and nurture the young people they choose."

H	Residency training	Late 30s	MAS, MD	K23	Dry	Asst adjunct prof (in res.)	K23, others

Having completed most of the research described in an earlier K-award application, H is reviewing the data and anxious about the applying for the RO1 necessary for joining the "real" UCSF faculty. With energy, skill, and tenacity, H's research focuses on implementing changes in treating and managing a complex, slow-moving, but life-threatening chronic disease.

J	Specialty fellowship	Late 30s	MD	K08	Wet	Asst prof (In res.)	K08, appl. for RO1

Although she lacked a PhD, J's quick wit and enthusiasm, combined with good judgment of leaders in a UCSF specialty fellowship training program, resulted in a promising lab project, an excellent mentor, and cobbled-together funds for salary. Hard work and productive research led to transfer from adjunct to in residence when J was 37. J is revising a first RO1 application and about to submit another. Success is not guaranteed, but prospects look good.

Legend to Table 9-6 opposite page.

and receiving K-awards. These investments have proved highly successful, as documented in recent surveys of two groups of awardees: (i) 155 K-awardees in the Department of Medicine (DOM), 2003-2012 (Table 9-4; *40*); (ii) 63 CTSI trainees in its K-Scholar Program, 2005-2011 (Table 9-5; *41*). The groups overlap (to a degree not precisely determined), but together represent ~180 awardees and 50% of all UCSF K-awardees during the years surveyed.

Of the 155 awardees in the DOM survey, 124 (80%) remained members of the UCSF faculty in 2013 (Table 9-4). As suggested by their types of K-award, about half of these were trained in "clinical" research, probably with a substantial dry-lab component, while many or most of the other half were probably trained in wet-lab research. Ninety-nine of those still on the UCSF faculty (~80%) were supported by research grant dollars in 2013, including 50 (40%) supported by NIH grants. As would be expected, the early and late cohorts among them (whose K-awards began in 2003-2007 and 2010-2012, respectively) show a time-dependent transition from adjunct to in residence or clinical faculty status. Of the 30 individuals who left UCSF for jobs elsewhere, 24 (80%) remain in academia, and 19 are now associate professors (Table 9-4).

The 63 graduates who responded to the survey of CTSI's K-Scholars (Table 9-5) included 45 MDs (including four MD-PhDs), an additional 12 PhDs, and five with other doctoral degrees. At the time of the survey most were active in academia, with academic ranks that rose as years passed after they entered the program. Their ability to obtain research grants also increased: 96% of the oldest cohort had NIH RO1 (or equivalent) grants. In all cohorts, most spend substantial proportions of time in clinical and translational research, and publish results of their work at respectable rates. By every measure, a high proportion of K-Scholar program trainees became productive academics, with most of their research focused on patients. (This survey did not record how many respondents were still at UCSF vs. how many took jobs elsewhere.)

In summary, the bare facts in both surveys indicate that K-award training at UCSF produces productive scientists who make valuable contributions to the growth and quality of research in the clinical units responsible for their

Legend to Table 9-6 (oppposite):
These young clinician-scientists, interviewed by Henry Bourne, tell us how some K-awardees view their training experience. To help young physician-scientists speak frankly, the table does not reveal their names, genders, and specific research interests. Nonetheless, each un-named individual, from A to J, has read and approved both data and descriptions attributed to her or his code letter.
¶Abbreviations: appl., applicant; Asst, assistant; Assoc, associate; In res., in residence; Post-grad., post-graduate.

training. Those who depart for positions elsewhere prove similarly successful.

Personal interviews with nine recent UCSF K-awardees (Table 9-6) confirm this group's impressive quality and success. Before we discuss them further, however, a few caveats: the number of interviewees is too small to support strong inferences about all UCSF K-awardees; most interviewees were recommended to the authors by leaders of clinical units, so their quality may be better than the average (at least in their leaders' eyes). At best, the snapshot sketches in Table 9-6 add nuance to our picture of the K-awardees' experience at UCSF and suggest topics for further inquiry.

The nine interviewees are bright and hard-working, with ages ranging from 35 (the youngest) to a few years past 40. Seven are in the in residence series, including two associate professors and five assistant professors; two are adjunct assistant professors. In addition to K-grants, three have their own NIH RO1, and most enjoy additional support from private sources or another faculty member's NIH grant. Three conduct primarily dry-lab research, four conduct wet-lab experiments, and the remaining two take both approaches. All are MDs; four have PhDs also, and two have Master's degrees. Eight came to UCSF years before the K-award (one as a medical student, three for residency training, four for specialty fellowships). Five are male, four female.

Transition from dependent status (K-award only) to RO1 funding— "the gold standard," one termed it—marks independent "full faculty" status. The interviewees in Table 9-6 recognize the uncertainty and stress surrounding this transition, but handle it differently. At one end of the spectrum, Dr. B— explicitly rejecting second-tier adjunct status—transferred directly into the UCSF faculty from training elsewhere, with an RO1 and a K08 obtained soon after arrival. Dr. A, blessed with good mentors and committed to a specific patient population, moved steadily from one grant to another, and now has an RO1. Near the spectrum's middle, Drs. J and H see real difficulties ahead but feel reasonably sure they can be managed: J, who never got a PhD degree, nonetheless appears on the verge of getting RO1 support for wet-lab projects; worried about the RO1 transition, H pushes a hard project forward with great enthusiasm and energy. At the spectrum's other end, Dr. C fears a faculty appointment is an unlikely outcome for a hard struggle mired in a "pyramid scheme," while Dr. F appears a bit discouraged and not firmly committed to her/his project. In sum, their experience and prospects are those expected for six smart young people competing in a difficult race to a worthwhile goal.

The three remaining interviewees, Drs. D, G, and E, raise a question that merits further exploration. A steady, thoughtful MD-PhD who has become a productive clinician-scientist with able and helpful research colleagues, Dr. D sorely misses belonging to a broadly interactive scientific community and finds the unrelenting demands on an assistant professor at UCSF "very isolating." Dr. G, also an MD-PhD, feels distinctly uneasy about pursuing science in an environment full of intense, able, almost "manic" clinicians whose work pays part of G's salary; G harshly criticizes relative unwillingness of clinical department leaders to judge and champion research of young scientists in their departments. The third, Dr. E, has successfully applied for an RO1 grant but expresses anger at being immersed in a small faculty enclave (in a large clinical division) whose other members are (she/he feels) indifferent to research.

In different ways, these three individuals feel afflicted by scientific isolation, and hunger for a community that shares intense commitment to science. Their perceived plights beg a relevant question: Is scientific isolation likely to accelerate or hinder scientific discovery? Nowadays, truly innovative science often takes place in communities that obsessively exchange scientific ideas and questions. Similarly, superb scientists seek environments that foster communication and provide ready access to new notions and facts. On the other hand, three modestly anomalous interviews may not constitute a real trend, but could instead reflect random chance or bias (42). Because the question itself remains significant, Chapter 10 will return to it.

Perspective

This chapter shows gratifying success of research in UCSF's clinical departments, documented by rapid and continued growth of external funding, significant scientific advances, and attraction and training of excellent clinician-scientist colleagues. Most strikingly, these successes were achieved in the face of real difficulties, by subtle jiu-jitsu that converts formidable obstacles into substantial advantages (Table 9-7). The jiu-jitsu magic merits further scrutiny, although its triumphs have not resolved every issue.

Jiu-jitsu triumphs. One example is the predominantly bottom-up governance of research in clinical departments, which reflects their relative autonomy in hiring faculty and financial control over many endowments, as well as professional fees earned by their faculties' clinical service. One might predict that relative lack of top-down prescriptive leadership would make it difficult for any large component (like clinical departments) of UCSF and other large biomedical centers to navigate successfully through the rapidly changing external difficulties, fiscal and otherwise, of the past two decades. Observations by a recent newcomer to the UCSF faculty, Jennifer Grandis, suggest that top-down prescriptive control was not necessary. As new director of the CTSI,

Table 9-7. UCSF Clinical Department Research:
Jiu-jitsu Triumphs Over Obstacles

Obstacles	Jiu-jitsu: obstacles = advantages
Bottom-up governance: lack of top-down control could weaken response to unexpected stress	Creative departments and divisions free to test different solutions, turning on a dime when necessary
Dollar constraints	
Decreased public support constrains state & federal research funding	Increase private funding (foundations, collaboration with industry, philanthropy)
	Professional fee dollars (modest amounts)
Research costs grow (wet-lab especially)	Expand dry-lab approaches, with major assist from CTSI
Increasing need for external salary support	See soft-money salary as opportunity, not burden
Hard to grow faculty, owing to San Francisco cost of living & few young researchers willing to move	Expand K-awards to "audition" young faculty candidates Hire senior top guns from elsewhere

Grandis finds that UCSF differs from her former "hierarchical" academic environment, in which leaders exerted strong top-down supervision over most activities, to promote cooperation for the larger entity's benefit. In contrast, at UCSF she finds a constellation of groups who focus on developing and sustaining the infrastructure and resources they need to succeed. She had not imagined such small, highly independent units could thrive, or conduct such innovative and exciting research (43). Indeed, it appears that compartmentation into separate clinical specialties provides opportunities for investigators to ask and answer innovative questions, as another faculty member suggests (24). UCSF's clinical departments and their divisions may often have mounted faster and more creative responses to rapidly changing challenges than would have been possible for larger, less mobile entities like the School of Medicine or UCSF itself.

The most dramatic challenges to research in clinical departments were tight fiscal constraints from decreased SEAs and flat-lined NIH budgets (beginning, respectively, in the 1990s and in 2004. In less straitened years, SEA dollars paid partial salary to a few ladder-rank faculty and salaries of some administrative personnel, and NIH grants were easier to tap for sponsored salaries. Forced to make do with less of both, clinical units turned to two fund sources: (i) professional fee income, which served as a lubricant, in modest amounts, to defend against small fiscal challenges to the research mission; (ii) private funding sources from foundations and philanthropic donors, endowment gifts, projects in collaboration with (or funded by) drug companies and others, and clinical trials. Without the funds garnered by these strenuous jiu-jitsu moves, research in clinical departments would have been severely curtailed.

In addition to shortfalls in research funding, increases in actual costs of research caused problems for every investigator, but especially for wet-lab researchers who had to pay students, postdocs, and technicians, and for technical instruments and care of animals. Clinical departments recouped some losses by further increasing their dry-lab research efforts, which do not involve animals or very expensive equipment. This jui-jitsu was strengthened by NIH's swerve toward translational research and generous CTSI grants (UCSF's first began in 2006) that trained more dry-lab investigators.

As SEAs waned, a third fiscal challenge was to increase contributions from sponsored research funds to investigators' salaries. The clinical departments' tradition of piecing faculty salaries together from clinical and grant money helped them to exploit "soft-money" salaries as opportunities, rather than suffer them as burdens.

Another major challenge to the research mission of clinical departments was to "grow" more clinician-researchers. The task was made harder by stiff competition for talented young people from research centers in cities where living costs are less, by the long period of training for people who wished to become first-rate researchers as well as skilled physicians, and by the clinician-researchers' habit of staying where they were trained. Here UCSF's effective jiu-jitsu strategy was to invest heavily into expanding training of K-awardees as an audition process for faculty candidates. Beginning just before the 21st century, UCSF persuaded excellent residents and fellows to apply to the NIH's expanding K-award program. The high dollar cost of supplementing K-awardees' salaries, paid over many years, added ~200 clinician-scientists to UCSF's faculty, and train dozens more who conduct research elsewhere. As many as 50% of the new faculty may be dry-lab researchers.

In addition to K-awardees, UCSF's clinical departments hired in the past 15 years a substantial number of "top gun" (often senior) researchers from other universities. This was a significant departure from previous practice: as one former UCSF leader used to say, "We don't wander looking for stars. UCSF makes its own stars, right here, from assistant professors." The actual number of top guns hired (a dozen, perhaps?) and, more important, their collective impact on the research mission are unknown.

Prevailing conventions in US medical schools sharply constrain UCSF's options for attracting first-class researchers to its clinical departments. The habit of recruiting most young faculty from home-grown K-awardees makes it hard to attract outstanding young scientists from other schools. Given this constraint, as a rational response to market forces the K-award system has worked very well for UCSF. It is far from perfect, however, because of the eat-what-you-kill principle and Darwinian selection of faculty from K-awardees who get an NIH research grant. These defects, as we perceive them at UCSF, probably affect most US medical schools in similar ways.

Growth also produces problems. Despite impressive successes, research in UCSF's clinical departments needs to learn how to manage internal conflicts and contradictions. The foremost problem: reliance on relentless expansion as the principal—or perhaps only—strategy for guiding development of clinical research and the entire clinical enterprise. Expansion can also generate serious long-term risks. If changing circumstances were to make it impossible for growth to continue at its former rate, its slowing or cessation could severely damage whatever has already been accomplished. Worse, expansion tends to blind its adherents to problems that accompany vast size of any institution or business, including a university. In particular, UCSF's bottom-up governance allows the clinical enterprise to be driven by internal momentum and decisions of department chairs and division chiefs. Lack of power over hiring clinicians, severely limits the abilities of the chancellor and medical school dean to guide or control growth. Uncontrolled growth of research in clinical departments, driven mainly by growth of the clinical enterprise itself, may not be healthy, especially in view of the federal government's stagnant commitment to supporting high quality investigation. While leaders may count on increased clinical revenues to provide extra dollars to nourish research and other academic missions, a clinical enterprise indifferent to its effects on UCSF's other missions could limit access to those dollars.

Moreover, sheer size also expands facilities needed for both clinical and academic activities, leading to geographic separations that limit interactions among clinician-researchers, and with basic scientists. As remedies, UCSF has tried well-designed websites, CTSI, and sincere exhortation without conspicuous success. Larger size also makes it harder to judge and groom young scientists for faculty positions, by limiting commitment to mentoring, training, and evaluating the young (and replacing that commitment with the eat-what-you-kill principle and Darwinian selection). Will such strategies preserve and promote creative and innovative research?

Other problems may not be traceable entirely to large size, but size does not make their resolution easier. Some of these include:

1. Increasing construction and maintenance costs of wet-lab facilities may weaken clinical departments' ardor for recruiting and supporting biologically-oriented investigators. As clinical growth continues, will

departments and divisions reduce their commitment to understanding mechanisms of disease and therapy?

2. The silo problem. Some clinical specialty silos promote good mentoring; others do not. Silos appear to hinder interaction and collaboration among wet-lab or dry-lab researchers in separate units, between clinician-scientists and basic science department faculty, and between dry-lab and wet-lab researchers. Is anyone paying attention?

3. "Soft-money" contributions from sponsored projects to faculty researchers' salaries continue to grow, despite funding shortfalls and NIH salary caps, but may deter young clinician-scientists from conducting innovative research.

4. With drive and ingenuity, clinician-investigators garnered more private research funding as NIH dollars declined. Still, philanthropy can focus on narrow goals, industrial sponsors may specify conclusions to be drawn from experiments, and both pay lower indirect costs. Can UCSF manage such pitfalls to preserve ardor for tackling difficult scientific problems and producing innovative new knowledge?

Each of these hazards shares with the others closely related dilemmas: (i) how to ensure uniform high quality in a large institution that expands in response to external pressures indifferent to its core missions; (ii) how to prevent remedies from being hindered by excessive size, widely separated silos, and bottom-up governance; (iii) growing size, per se, does not provide a truly sustainable funding model for clinical department research in the long term, as indicated by soft-money as the prevailing salary source, and uneasiness about the extent to which clinical income should help to finance research. In this Rubik's cube each dilemma, issue, or remedy impinges on and constrains the others, and the cube cannot be solved by rhetorical flourishes and ruthless edicts. Instead, chapter 10 will propose complementary approaches, compromises, and experimental measures designed to move separate parts of the cube in the right direction.

Chapter 10

Skies uncertain as a child's bottom: Proposals for change

This book set out to perform three tasks. The preceding nine chapters were devoted to the first two: (i) to serve as a primer for readers who want to learn how and where research dollars flow in a large center devoted to academic biomedical research; (ii) to show, in broad terms, how distribution of resources within such a center guides and constrains investigators' goals and training of young scientists. The present (and last) chapter focuses on the third—and most difficult—task: to examine the prospects for UCSF's future research enterprise and propose tentative approaches to improve those prospects. Although the book focuses primarily on research at UCSF, readers better acquainted with other research centers will have already recognized many underlying problems shared by most of these centers. Indeed, at least 20 large academic biomedical institutions in the US share triumphs and difficulties very similar to those we have described at UCSF. Each differs in details from the others, but the underlying challenges closely resemble those at UCSF, and present similar arrays of difficult choices. Thus an assessment of UCSF's problems—and perhaps even proposals for handling them—may prove useful to academic scientists and leaders elsewhere. This chapter's primary goal is to ensure that these problems are recognized, investigated, and debated—and then, if necessary, carefully managed. Although none of the dangers requires emergency intervention, ignoring them could pose real dangers, and paying attention now may prevent later troubles.

By any measure, UCSF has enjoyed remarkable success for almost six decades. Successes in all its missions—patient care, education, and research—resulted from a fortunate combination of influences (Table 10-1), including an attractive city, bottom-up institutional governance, a fast-growing clinical enterprise of high quality, first-rate science, and agile handling of change and adversity. In the 21st century, UCSF's research community is rich in cultural

Table 10-1. Research at UCSF: Successes and Assets

Research successes and assets	See chapter(s)
1. Fifty years of steady growth in external funding allowed new laboratories to make major discoveries and advances	1, 7-9
2. Rapid growth in size, wealth, and quality of clinical enterprise helps to defray research costs	1, 7-9
3. Bottom-up governance, especially in clinical departments, permits separate growth of foci for independent, original research and nurture for nurturing young talent, especially in clinical departments	9
4. Abundant cultural capital: traditions of collaboration and nurturing young scientists, standard of excellence, scientific discovery	7-9
5. Effective responses to change, since late 1970s, include: diverse, well integrated graduate programs; growing dollar support despite government cutbacks; K-awards develop superb young scientists	4-9
6. Location in a city that attracts smart, adventurous people	1, 7-9
Consequently:	
7. UCSF researchers are numerous, broadly focused, and excellent	

capital, with a critical mass of excellent investigators, but external problems (Table 10-2) threaten its ability to exploit exciting opportunities—greater today than ever—for biomedical discovery and innovative advances in health care. This last chapter will not dwell on triumphs, which are amply recounted in earlier chapters. Instead, here we focus on problems and challenges that need attention, and propose institutional responses that may help to overcome them.

We begin by listing major problems we see for research at UCSF and similar institutions. Some problems are large in scope, while others affect separate elements of the research community; all, however, are complex and multifaceted:

1. Academic health centers already face financial difficulties in sustaining their academic missions, especially research. The difficulties are unlikely to lessen soon.

2. Researchers in basic science departments are severely constrained by needing to pay ever-larger fractions of their salaries from "soft money"—that is, from research grants—and by the fact that the names and teaching responsibilities of their departments bear little relation to their scientific goals or subjects they teach.

3. Clinical department researchers face similar constraints from soft-money salaries.

Table 10-2. Research at UCSF: External Problems, Challenges

	Chapters
1. Competition against other large health centers drives growth of UCSF's hospitals, with major effects (good and bad) on research	1, 9
2. Diminishing willingness of US citizens and their governments to pay for research and education	1, 2
2. Decreased federal research funding (in constant dollars)	1, 3, 7-9
3. Decreased state support for faculty salaries and research facilities	1, 2, 7-9
4. Soaring cost of living in San Francisco	7-9
5. Stiff competition (from private universities and state campuses with many students) for students, researchers, grants, and philanthropy	6, 7-9
6. Nation-wide academic policies hinder efforts to change scientific training, lab organization, or faculty evaluation and salaries at UCSF	7-9
These problems threaten UCSF's ability to promote transformative discovery and devise innovative ways to treat and prevent disease.	

4. Academic silos narrow the focus of many investigators and limit their interactions with scientific colleagues.

5. Compared to their elders, young biomedical researchers are disproportionately disadvantaged with respect to salary, grant awards, and research opportunities.

6. Rapid clinical expansion and sheer size of biomedical centers encourage arbitrary quantitative criteria for research excellence that ignore creativity, innovation, and impact.

Before we describe specific proposals, caveats are in order. First, four of our five proposals focus primarily on research. Second, several of these proposals resemble those proposed by others. Third, none of the proposals guarantees success, owing to potential fatal flaws we did not detect, incorrect diagnoses of underlying problems, and the sheer unpredictability of future events. Fourth, as readers will quickly realize, these proposals are not directly keyed to the six problems listed above, because each problem intertwines with others. Rather than conjure neat (but imaginary) "fixes" for mega-problems, we proffer specific measures to ameliorate complex effects that reflect multiple causes; some of those causes cannot be tackled directly. If readers find our diagnoses and proposals wrong or inadequate, we urge them to devise their own.

Proposal 1. A substantial General Endowment for UCSF

For decades, UCSF's inherited anti-authoritarian ethos and abundant external resources allowed semi-independent entities, large and small, to grow in directions and at rates determined by opportunity, energy, and creativity; freedom from repressive authority made it possible for individuals and groups to develop agile, fast-moving projects. As we have seen, control of most key resources—including space (chapters 4 and 7); many revenue sources (e.g., grants and clinical professional fees; chapters 1-3, 7-9); and endowment dollars (chapter 4)—is distributed preferentially to individuals (e.g., salary endowments), departments, and divisions, relative to deans or the Chancellor's office. This preferential distribution of power and autonomy to individuals and semi-independent units can hinder responses to challenges like those listed in Table 10-2, which require concerted action by many units at once.

Unable to wrest substantial monetary resources from the state, existing endowments, or clinical revenues, deans and chancellors have a single alternative: philanthropy. The Chancellor's "Infrastructure and Operations Fund" (IOF; chapter 2) squeezes some dollars from UCSF's other endowments; while some of these dollars will be needed to maintain fund-raising efforts that attract them, yearly increases of $17M or more in the Chancellor's endowment payout will help to stabilize central administration and maintain ongoing programs over the next decade.

Over and above the IOF, however, reinforcing UCSF's top-down ability to respond to external challenges absolutely requires the kind of financial support and stability provided by a robust General Endowment, like those available to many private institutions, but lacking at UCSF. The institution's leaders have not actively sought donations to a substantial General Endowment for UCSF, but should do so now, for powerful negative and positive reasons. On the negative side, as previous chapters show, at UCSF in the 21st century research is inherently not sustainable from multiple available resources—e.g., state and federal government, collaborations with profit-driven private companies, or margins earned by the clinical enterprise. Moreover, for a Campus without undergraduates, tuition and fees cannot begin to suffice. None of these resources are themselves stable and likely to increase sufficiently over the short or long term; while clinical revenues may appear more reliable, they are already inadequate to foot the research bills, and future health care funding remains in flux, to say the least.

The positive reason for a General Endowment: unexpected clinical margins, accumulated or projected in fiscal years 2015-2017, provide several tens of millions of dollars (chapter 5) to nucleate such an endowment. Clinical largesse may wax or wane thereafter, like the fat and lean kine in a Pharaoh's dream (*1*), but within a few decades UCSF's reputation and the energy of its development office—plus a change of heart among UCSF's leaders—could increase the General Endowment's principal to as much as ~$500M, producing annual payouts of ~$18-25M. No one can know what the future holds, but if UCSF had started to accumulate a General Endowment 30 years ago, by now the principal would come to several hundred million dollars—enough to prove immensely useful for strategic purposes.

Obvious potential benefits of such a General Endowment include enhanced fiscal stability, funds for flexible responses to stormy future economic conditions, and repairing (albeit only in part) effects of unrelenting cuts in state educational support over the past 25 years. In addition, such an endowment may prove essential for maintaining and enhancing UCSF's capacity for innovative academic missions, from training researchers and clinicians to fostering world-class research.

Proposal 2. A Basic Science Division to replace basic science departments

Many researchers in UCSF's basic science departments are discouraged by a slowly worsening drought of inflation-corrected research grant dollars from NIH (for them, a 10+% decrease over 10 years, while the NIH budget diminished by 22%; chapter 7), and by increasing pressure to support large fractions of their own salaries from grants (chapters 7 and 8; see proposal 3, below). They also feel neglected: deans and the Chancellor, they feel, focus more and more attention on clinical expansion and its attendant problems, and less on erstwhile star researchers in basic science.

This malaise may be a relic of a governance scheme that has become irrelevant: UCSF's basic science departments form a congeries of fossil silos inherited from earlier decades, when department names referred to subjects taught to professional students. Consequently, 112 researchers who currently receive sponsored funds (*2*) are distributed among eight basic science departments in three Schools, where they pursue administratively unconnected agendas, rather than negotiating ways to handle their common problems with deans and chancellors. We propose a logical merger of these 112 faculty into a Basic Science Division (BSD), replacing the eight fossil silos with a half-dozen sections (not fossil remnants) within the BSD; sections could represent research disciplines, graduate programs, or—in order to foster communication across disciplines—by random assignment or location within UCSF.

The BSD would take primary responsibility for managing material resources, while a quasi-federal arrangement would allow the BSD and sections to share control of academic appointments, rank, obligations, and privileges. The BSD's chief would be appointed by the Chancellor and deans of the three schools whose faculty now belong to basic science departments. This chief, with a steering committee of faculty and section chairs (3), would control distribution of faculty salary contributions from UCSF, faculty start-up packages, space, renovation and construction of facilities, human resources, post-award grant administration, and salaries for the sections' administrative staff. Sections would contain approximately equal numbers of faculty slots (subject to initial negotiations and deans' discretion), conduct searches for new faculty, vote on appointments and promotions, negotiate salaries, and approve space assignments. All section decisions would require approval and funds from the BSD chief and steering committee, and the BSD chief would be a member of the Chancellor's Executive Cabinet (see chapter 5). Overall, such an arrangement would facilitate negotiations between leaders and basic science faculty and better align key administrative decisions with needs of the basic science community.

This short account cannot do justice to all complications and difficulties the new arrangement may entail. The knottiest of these is identifying which basic scientists should be included in the BSD, and which high official(s) should oversee it. We propose that the BSD include all 112 members of UCSF's basic science departments (2). In FY 2014, only 58 (barely more than half) of these received sponsored dollars (see Table 8-2 and reference 4) through departments in the School of Medicine (Anatomy, Biochemistry and Biophysics, Cellular and Molecular Pharmacology, Microbiology and Immunology, and Physiology), while 54 received their sponsored funds through the Schools of Pharmacy (Pharmaceutical Chemistry and Bioengineering and Therapeutic Sciences) and Dentistry (Cell and Tissue Biology). A few faculty with primary appointments in basic science departments received their sponsored funds through ORUs, and are counted within the 73 ORU scientists with sponsored funds (Table 8-2, and reference 4); the laboratories of these latter individuals are often located in ORU space. If the BSD (and perhaps its sections) were to include the 112 individuals whose sponsored funds come through academic departments in Medicine, Pharmacy, and Dentistry, the Division would operate across school boundaries, in collaboration with both the Chancellor and the Schools. Its faculty would be subject to the BSD's jurisdiction and rules—and, through their section and the BSD, to both their Schools and the Chancellor. Although by no means tidy, this solution has a clear precedent, UCSF's Graduate Division. Despite administrative difficulties, a BSD including faculty in multiple Schools presents critical advantages for research. Including researchers and departments from all three Schools would give the BSD more clout in negotiations and spread its benefits to a larger number of faculty. Most important, all BSD faculty would share common interests in wet-lab laboratories, fundamental biology, human biology, and pathogenesis of disease, and no present basic science department faculty would be left out.

Proposal 3. Targeted endowment(s) to reduce researchers' soft-money salaries

The widespread need of research faculty to earn large (and increasing) portions of their salaries from research grants poses grave threats to the integrity and quality of research. Such a need saps researchers' morale and makes them vulnerable to arbitrary decisions of external funders. It also attenuates their loyalty to one another and to their institution; reciprocally, an institution that pays only small fractions of salary to researchers is less likely to respect and care for them in other ways. Another threat is even more critical: for investigators who depend on each year's grant dollars to feed their families, risk of failure becomes unacceptable, reducing their willingness to tackle difficult questions or propose experiments that do. The inevitable tendency of soft money to sharpen the danger of small failures undermines the creativity and innovation that make first-rate research useful to citizens and patients.

Although UCSF and its competitor institutions recognize these dangers, the sheer size of their financial dilemma stymies effective responses. For example, UCSF could never make up for the annual $148M in salary plus benefits its researchers derived from external sources in FY2014, combined with the additional $60M in ICR that comes with that salary; together loss of both the sponsored salary support and the ICR would amount to a total of $208M (see chapter 3). Replacing that amount would require 5% annual payout from a (new) endowment of $4.16B (5)—effectively quenching all ardor for "fixing" (or even for trying to mitigate) the soft-money dilemma.

Our proposal is straightforward: UCSF should begin by mounting a deliberate effort to remedy soft money's worst consequences, by jump-starting an endowment—of, say, $80M rather than $4B—to target small but effective amounts of research support (Targeted Research Awards, or TRAs) to critical subgroups of important research faculty. TRA arithmetic might go something like this: a 5% payout from an endowment of $80M would earn ~$4M per year. Compared to $208M, $4M seems an insignificant sum, but compared to the zero dollars presently available it looks better: indeed, it could provide an average of $80,000 in hard money (or ~$62,000 in salary plus $18,000 In benefits) to 50 researchers every year. Where might 50 dollops of this size make the greatest possible difference to UCSF's research effort? First, let us identify faculty groups who should *not* receive these dollars, under at least four headings:

1. Because soft money salaries adversely affect researchers in both basic science and clinical departments (*6*), neither group should be exclusively targeted for TRAs.
2. TRA dollars should not go to senior researchers. If their research is first-rate, they will prosper in any case; the money is less likely to change other seniors' careers.
3. Deans, department chairs, or division chiefs already distribute abundant support from other sources, but should play no role in distributing TRAs.
4. Rather than support long-lasting professorships, TRAs should be awarded to faculty for limited periods that can make a genuine difference to their subsequent careers.

Together these restrictions help to assure that no choices to target TRAs to a specific faculty subset should bolster strength of existing academic silos, preserve advantages of older as compared to younger faculty, or make it harder for the institution to sustain its research mission over the long term. (Nor should a TRA ever serve as a substitute for support already supplied through traditional department channels.) Rather than depend on chairs and existing leaders to distribute payouts from the TRA endowment, communities of basic science department faculty and clinician-scientists can devise their own criteria for TRA awards to their members. For instance, payouts from $40M of the TRA endowment could pay an extra $75,000 per year to every ladder rank basic science faculty member promoted to the rank of associate professor, for a six-year period or until she/he is promoted to full professor (*7*). Such mid-career funding boosts can accelerate innovative advances that will drive subsequent research careers.

UCSF's Department of Medicine (DOM) just announced an In Residence Associate Professor Support (IRAPS) program (*8*) designed to augment institution-supplied salary for its research-focused associate professors in residence by $50,000 per year. Thus the DOM is betting that mid-career researchers will benefit most from the supplement, which will relieve them of the need to divert a similar amount of dollars (in salary plus benefits) from sponsored projects. While one large silo, the DOM, was able to commit enough dollars to pay this institutional supplement for all its in residence researchers at the level of associate professor, it is not clear that all clinical departments will be able to follow suit. In light of this recent development, the proposed TRA program would presumably specify that its dollars not replace supplementary institutional dollars already provided by a department; as noted above, communities of basic science department faculty and clinician-scientist faculty would devise their own criteria for choosing the subset of researcher faculty members to receive TRA dollars.

For prospective philanthropists, the proposed TRA endowment combines academic innovation with an attractive research goal, fundamental biological investigation. Additional advantages of TRAs for basic scientists, clinician-researchers, and UCSF itself might include: research faculty participation in a broad coalition unconstrained by silos, chairs, and division chiefs; using UCSF's persuasive faculty to help attract endowment dollars that can directly improve their colleagues' careers and their scientific environment; focusing UCSF and its entire scientific community on their mutual responsibilities for both academic change and research. Similar principles should apply to all of UCSF's large endowments and philanthropic gifts (see Box 10-1).

Would the TRA endowment and the General Endowment (proposed above) compete against each other for philanthropic support? Although we are not expert seekers of philanthropic dollars, we strongly suspect the answer is yes. Still, proper management can moderate the intensity of that competition and reduce its potential detriments. Different donors may prefer the two endowments' distinct purposes: one aimed at benefitting all UCSF's missions, another targeted to a specific problem that threatens innovative research. It might also be useful to link the two endowments, supporting TRAs from a Fund Functioning as Endowment (FFE; see chapters 2 and 4), as a distinct component of General Endowment, which would constitute a permanent but administratively flexible support for the entire institution.

Proposal 4. Redress disproportionate advantages of seniority vs. youth

Many young UCSF researchers feel their progress is slower than it should be, and disproportionately so in comparison to senior faculty. Available records did not allow us to determine whether young UCSF faculty receive propor-

Box 10-1. Endowment dollars can accelerate academic change

Large endowments to UCSF often focus on providing benefits to a single worthy element of a larger mission—the research program of a small subset of faculty, students of this or that School or program, care of a particular disease or a particular class of patients. Chapter 2 discussed one such case: a $30M gift, to which UCSF added a similar sum from one of its own FFEs, was targeted to support for graduate students in laboratories of its faculty. The cause was eminently worthy, and the dollars have certainly relieved hard-pressed graduate programs and researchers from part of the financial burden of supporting graduate students (to a large extent, from research grants). Faculty researchers, along with the graduate division and academic leaders, failed to ask a crucial question, however: whether, in addition to relieving some of the costs, the endowment money could be used to enhance the quality of graduate education at UCSF (9). In our view, UCSF's leaders, its faculty, and its development office, should *never* assume that lack of dollars is the only defect an endowment can or should correct; instead, they should be constantly alert to the possibility of leveraging a large gifts to produce necessary academic change. To make this happen, UCSF's leaders would have to adopt this approach and deliberately apply it as often as possible.

tionately less sponsored funds than in the past, but the national data is crystal-clear: from 1980 to 2006, federal grant funding shifted substantially away from US medical school faculty in their thirties and toward senior investigators in their late fifties and sixties (*10*). The shift continues: *US PIs older than 60 received 12% of NIH research project grant dollars in 1998, vs. 28% in 2014 (11)*. No magic can have rescued UCSF's young faculty from this strong trend.

Similar pressures weigh on biomedical research trainees (graduate students and postdocs) and young people seeking their first faculty research position (chapters 8 and 9). At every level, pressures on the young reflect fierce competition for volatile (and diminishing) federal funds, decreased state support for faculty salaries, long scientific training, and—especially in San Francisco—higher costs for housing and for educating children (chapters 1, 2, and 6-9). PhD students, postdoctoral scholars, and MDs or MD-PhDs with K-awards worry about long years of training and financial difficulties of starting a family. Supporting much of their salary from grants, young basic science faculty are troubled to find that their seniors often pay lower mortgages and renew their grants more easily. Sharing those worries, young clinician-researchers may also feel trapped in small enclaves, where they depend on often-arbitrary Darwinian selection by granting agencies while their seniors pay substantial portions of large salaries from endowments and large clinical incomes. Local interventions to mitigate these problems will vary, depending upon whether the young scientists are being trained, looking for their first faculty positions, or growing their labs for the first time.

In addition to learning how to do research, graduate students, PhD post-docs, and MDs or MD-PhDs all face two severe problems: financial difficulties of living (and sometimes starting a family) in San Francisco, and/or the long duration of their training. UCSF is working actively to provide affordable housing for trainees (see chapter 8), but has not streamlined or accelerated their scientific training. If bright young people keep coming into biomedical research, institutions will not offer shorter training paths to attract trainees. But for graduate students this attitude is short-sighted (see chapter 8), because training that may not be necessary delays their careers by about two years. One US graduate program reduced time-to-PhD-degree by 1.5-2 years and preserved its graduates' competitive edge (12). UCSF could easily fund a small experiment to ask whether PhDs who graduate in 4.5 years get research jobs comparable to those of graduates whose training lasts for 6-7 years (12). If so, students would flock to programs that offer a better chance of becoming scientists two years sooner. Other complications can be managed (13).

As K-awardees, young clinician-scientists must survive years of work in a faculty member's laboratory before NIH's Darwinian competition decides whether or not they get an RO1 (chapter 9). The notion that NIH reviewers are better winnowers than UCSF's established clinician-researchers may be correct, but only if the latter are simply too busy or too lazy to do a good job. And the K-award-to-obligatory-RO1-award ordeal prevails in part because clinical departments and divisions prefer not to invest time or money in scientists chosen by supra-departmental or supra-divisional (SD/SC) consortiums, because the chosen candidates may join enclaves they do not control. Nonetheless, a committee of first-rate UCSF clinician-researchers could certainly choose faculty better than the NIH does, providing they can meet the candidate scientists and hear their research seminars. On a small scale, UCSF's clinical departments are probably rich enough to devise and conduct an experiment to ask whether a well-constituted SD/SC search committee can find, and UCSF can attract, one superb clinician-scientist each year, chosen from both visiting and local applicants. Over 10 years, four will probably become superb researchers, and most of the others will perform excellent research—a batting average comparable to that established by UCSF's basic science departments for decades. This experiment is worth a try.

At a larger scale, of course, as compared to established older faculty, young faculty clearly find it harder to obtain and maintain research funding. This is an excellent rationale for helping the best of these young people by supplementing their salary and grants with TRAs, as described above. The total number of available dollars probably will not suffice to help every worthy young clinician-scientist in early years of faculty service. If so, it will be crucial—as a genuine contribution to salutary academic change—that TRA recipients be chosen by SD/SC committees, and *not* by barter/bargain negotiations among chairs and division chiefs.

Finally, it is worth repeating that our limited, local proposals may help young scientists who represent the future of research, but cannot relieve the underlying external pressures responsible for relative disadvantages of young vs. older scientists: the competition for scarce research support, weak state support, long scientific training, and higher living costs. We do, however, urge senior scientists to remember when their own fledgling efforts were supported by their seniors' generosity and by a system less severely stressed than it has become in the early 21st century.

Proposal 5. Funds functioning as endowments to foster silo-bridging research

Creativity thrives when scientists exchange ideas freely, compare and share goals and technologies, and combine competition with collaboration. Squeezing research into silos damps creativity by hindering communication. Consider three UCSF examples:

1. *Intellectual separation.* When the Department of Biochemistry and Biophysics (B&B) regenerated its research in the 1970s, faculty in its turreted redoubts began to regard other basic science departments as entities justified only by fulfilling medical students' need to learn their subjects. The DNA revolution of the 1980s, however, converted B&B and the other basic science departments into a thriving research syncytium (13), and by the 21st century their former intellectual silos had become withered husks, ready to blow away (see Proposal 1, above).

2. *Geographic separation.* Once the basic sciences crossed the Bay to return to San Francisco in the late 1950s, clinical department chairs played major roles in fostering regeneration of research in basic science departments

(13). But now basic science departments are more isolated from the rest of UCSF than ever before, partly owing to their nearly complete relocation from Parnassus to Mission Bay in 2003.

3. *Administrative separation, by clinical specialty.* Clinician-researchers receive scientific training, but their medical subspecialty specifies which department or division will recruit them to join the faculty. In combination with the size of the clinical enterprise, dependence on dollars earned by delivering specialty care separates researchers into silos that rarely communicate with denizens of other silos.

Recognizing that multiple small silos are not optimal ways to organize research, deans and chancellors have tried to construct bridges between investigators of basic science and clinical departments, or among scientists in different clinical units. In the latter regard, such efforts—e.g., the Biomedical Sciences Graduate Program (centered at Parnassus), the CTSI, interdisciplinary seminar series, and modest research support awarded to collaborations involving two or more silos (see chapters 7-9)—have not been very effective, because small dollops of money and seminars are no match for proximity, financial support from an administrative unit, or co-participation in clinical care.

Silos will certainly always be with us, partly as convenient administrative tools, and also because their protection can sometimes encourage creativity within small groups. Still, it appears clear to us and to many researchers, that poor communication between large silos (e.g., basic science and clinical departments) wastes opportunities for collaboration, while confinement within a small silo (e.g., a small division in a clinical department) can (and sometimes does) isolate and desiccate fertile minds.

Accordingly, we propose that deans and chancellors cooperate with faculty to combat that isolation and desiccation by setting up small FFEs (discussed in chapters 2 and 4) to support research by groups of faculty who reside in more than one department or division. This approach can be usefully fungible, in that endowment dollars for X research can open many different kinds of research opportunity: depending on X, such dollars could jumpstart nascent research, advance ongoing research, or bring disparate groups together to achieve shared long-term goals. Ideally, a thoughtful, imaginative dean could encourage such approaches by detecting and helping small nascent communities of scattered researchers who have already had some success in coordinating their efforts with those of scientists in other silos *(15)*. While existing silos are loath to contribute dollars and effort to hoist researchers out of old silos and stuff them into a new one, our imaginative dean would begin by enlisting help from a leader in the small initial group, giving the imaginary consortium a name (X, for "extraordinary"), and supporting X on a jump-start shoestring)—i.e., a small office and a part-time secretary (funded, perhaps, by the General Endowment envisioned in Proposal 1).

Then comes the pivotal next step: UCSF's development office, with a dollop of publicity and help from persuasive researchers in the initial group, launches a modest campaign to attract philanthropic dollars to support X. If the campaign produces $25M for the new FFE's principal, the ~$1.25M annual payout can: help X grow in directions guided by its researchers and the dean who started the campaign; circumvent UCSF's formidable size by opening opportunities for X's researchers to find expert collaborators in the institution; preserve the researchers' relations to their original silos; and, finally, encourage other nascent research groups to transcend their silo-bound fates by cooperating with leaders to form consortiums Y and Z. If the project either achieves its goal or proves unsuccessful within a pre-set period (15 years or so), the dean would presumably retain the original FFE and could apply it to a different project.

Can UCSF harness its clinical growth to sustain research?

We pose that critical question in lieu of offering a concrete proposal for handling three difficult and closely related problems: clinical expansion, the immense size of an institution like UCSF, and the (often unrecognized) near-impossibility of sustaining creative research by relying on the "margin" (aka profit) of a clinical enterprise.

We begin with a straightforward fact: since the 1960s, UCSF's clinical enterprise has expanded steadily, at a rate twice as fast as the growth of its academic Campus (chapters 1, 7, and 9). As that growth waxed even more exuberant over the past 25 years, UCSF earned a glowing reputation for first-rate clinical care across a broad spectrum of diseases and technical advances, and delivered much-needed care to vulnerable populations in San Francisco and the third world. These achievements attracted bright students, many patients, innovative faculty, technology entrepreneurs, and philanthropists, as well as research funds from federal and private sources. Now, as UCSF Health merges with Bay Area hospitals and partners with primary care and other delivers of health care, the clinical enterprise is projected to grow even faster: revenues of the combined clinical-academic enterprise will soon surpass $6B per year—one third greater than revenues in FY2014, the index year chosen for this book.

The rationale for this accelerated clinical expansion: simple survival. In the rapidly consolidating US health care industry, the institution's clinics and hospitals cannot "successfully vie for patients and contracts" without owning or partnering with health-care delivery systems "whose cost structures are lower than [UCSF's] academic medical center" (16). We have no reason to doubt this alarming survival rationale, but this book's focus prompts us to pose a critical question: can further expansion of the clinical enterprise preserve the quality of UCSF's research mission? The proffered answer, in 2015, is yes: "[R]evenue from UCSF Health is, by far, the largest source of flexible dollars that we use [for many purposes,] . . . and to support our researchers (with the cuts in NIH funding over the past decade, even successful researchers can no longer fully support themselves without help) . . . ." (16) Note, however, that this "yes" makes no claim that clinical revenue dollars will *suffice* to maintain research at UCSF.

Indeed, blunt truths cast serious doubt on any positive answer to our question. First, most of the increased clinical revenue from affiliating with additional hospitals and physicians does not and cannot provide "flexible dollars" to support researchers—or any mission beyond maintaining the health care delivery systems required to maintain patient volume and contracts for UCSF's academic medical center. More clinicians and patients generate needs for ever-greater capital investment in buildings, offices, and hospital facilities, plus pressing needs for housing more faculty, staff, and students. Second, the medical center's revenues are already proving inadequate to subsidize research in either basic science or clinical departments at levels they clearly need. So far, no "business model" for research at UCSF has shown how clinical revenues can sustain it by paying the unrecovered indirect costs of research for the next 20 years. Even smoke and mirrors cannot produce such a business model, because clinical revenues are unlikely to grow fast enough in the foreseeable future to pay all those costs. The upshot: academic research cannot be sustained without strong support from government and philanthropy.

A third blunt truth is harder: although it may prove essential for UCSF's future, clinical expansion inexorably diverts much-needed academic attention from teaching and research toward the myriad critical issues that arise in building more medical offices and clinical facilities and forging complex agreements, contracts, mergers, and affiliations. Rapid responses to opportunities or threats require unrelenting energy and attention, so chancellors, deans, department chairs, division chiefs, and faculty necessarily focus less energy, skills, and attention on financially smaller, less alluring academic challenges, which often call for long-term remedies that cannot work without continuing determination and efforts of academic leaders, and their successors.

In addition to separating clinicians, researchers, and teachers into enclaves, UCSF's growing size nudges its missions to define goals and assess effects in numbers (of people, dollars, or assignable square feet), rather than on academic quality. A strong focus on quantity allows leaders to brag about UCSF's gargantuan research engine and massive health system, but tempts them to recruit high-profile senior figures in the laboratory and the clinic and attenuates their once strong commitment to judging the quality of research by investigators already present at UCSF. Examples: (i) emphasis on ICR/asf as a primary criterion for proper utilization of research space; (ii) allowing NIH's reviewers of RO1 grants to replace the local scientific community's judgment for deciding whether a young clinician-scientist should join the faculty (chapters 4, 8, and 9).

UCSF's leaders, not coincidentally, are the triumvirate that presides over UCSF Health (see Fig. 1-1b): Sam Hawgood, UCSF's Chancellor and Chair of the Health System; Mark Laret, the System's President and CEO; and Talmadge King, Jr., Vice Chancellor for Medical Affairs and Dean of the School of Medicine. With respect to the research mission, however, these thoughtful, able leaders appear so far not have confronted a daunting contradiction. On the one hand, clinical expansion will surely continue, owing to its own inexorable momentum, the strong belief that expansion is necessary for the institution's survival, and the fact that neither the Dean of Medicine nor the Chancellor possesses the necessary power to control clinical hires—power that is exerted by the Medical Center and clinical department chairs (see chapter 9). On the other hand, clinical growth not only poses its own dangers for research, but also—and more important—probably cannot supply enough support for research to make up for lost state and federal dollars.

Faced with this contradiction, what should UCSF's leaders do to make research a sustainable mission for their institution? Rather than offering a concrete proposal, we strongly urge that UCSF recognize this challenging contradiction and decide explicitly how, or even whether, to deal with it. Indeed, our greatest fear is that UCSF's leaders—especially those charged with stewardship of the Campus mission—will inadvertently fail to confront the contradiction. As stewards of the Campus, the Chancellor and the Dean of Medicine—along with the other UCSF Deans and most department chairs—correctly see themselves as exerting enormous effort and distributing many valuable dollars to support research, which they sincerely consider a critically important academic mission.

Nonetheless, it is fair to ask those leaders (and their predecessors and successors) to take a comprehensive view, with a perspective longer than the next few years, of prospects for research at UCSF. Such a view would compare what kind of institutional support research will deserve, vs. the support it is likely to receive—30-50 years hence. As we have seen, state and federal government, volatile and fickle even in their occasional bursts of generosity, offer ever-diminishing support for research; private industry pushes its own driving agenda; and philanthropy needs to be guided to think in terms of decades and half-centuries rather than quick fixes. Deleterious results are already apparent: researcher salaries have become dangerously "soft;" dollars are directed preferentially to silos and support senior faculty rather than broad collaborative projects; major responsibility for judging quality of young researchers has been transferred to external judges (e.g., at NIH); older investigators gradually accrue more and more power, autonomy, and research dollars; institutional support for recruiting, training, and fostering careers of young scientists becomes less stable; and working scientists (in both basic science and clinical departments) frequently complain that the institution focuses most of its attention elsewhere.

This book's introduction described a past half-century during which no academic health center could aspire to a national leadership role without a primary commitment to research. Indeed, UCSF made itself a national leader by its stewardship of biomedical research as the essential life-blood of the institution. Now, in sharp contrast, UCSF's stewards may fail to assess accurately the future prospects for its research mission. Such an assessment failure can produce unexpected and undesired long-term consequences. One such consequence might be to consign innovative research at UCSF, once valued as the institution's life-blood, to protracted entropic decline.

Alternatively, the institution's leaders could decide to undertake a careful and objective assessment of the prospects for funding a truly first-rate research enterprise over the coming 30-50 years. Such an assessment would not be an easy undertaking, but only in part because it would have to compete against expansion and its demands for attention of UCSF's leaders. Suppose, instead, that a genuinely hard-nosed assessment shows it is quite unlikely that UCSF's clinical enterprise and philanthropy can combine to support first-rate research over the long term: truly hard decisions would then become unavoidable. It would be lovely, of course, if that assessment were to indicate that UCSF can find a way to sustain vigorous, innovative research over the long run. If so, the successful model may require some combination of: deliberately contracting certain local research commitments in order to preserve others; copious and well-directed philanthropy; out-competing other academic centers for government support; judicious management of collaborations with the health-care industry; and extraordinary luck (one of UCSF's real specialties!). In any case, we strongly urge that such an assessment be made, soon.

These are tall orders indeed! Time will tell.

UCSF's future prospects

We began this book by highlighting UCSF's conflicts between extravagant hopes and harsh realities. Focusing almost exclusively on the institution's research mission, this chapter has proposed five potentially useful responses to today's realities: a General Endowment; a Basic Science Division; TRA endowment(s) to reduce soft-money salaries; measures to redress disadvantages of young vs. senior scientists; and FFEs to support silo-bridging research. As we warned at the outset, our proposals do not strike deep into the core of every danger UCSF faces. This is because many problems are external to UCSF and thus beyond its control, and core internal issues, like clinical expansion and long-term sustainability of research, are too complex and multifaceted to be tackled successfully by any proposals we dare to make.

While our proposals for UCSF may not precisely fit challenges familiar to readers whose academic homes are elsewhere, careful consideration will reveal similar dilemmas and suggest parallel proposals to deal with them. Whether or not UCSF and its denizens choose to ignore our proposals, the institution's momentum and internal strengths will keep it moving forward, nonetheless. We think our proposals are worth considering because they harness UCSF's capacity for imaginative and effective responses to troubles and crises, some of which were harder to handle than those it faces today. The first such response, 50 years ago, ousted a chancellor in order to establish research as a guiding mission (14). Others include effective handling of San Francisco's sudden AIDS epidemic in the 1980s (17); converting department-based PhD training into multi-disciplinary biomedical graduate programs (14); and the hospitalist strategy to improve in-patient care in large medical centers (18). Today no one can predict what will happen to the US medical care system, academic biomedicine, research funding, or UCSF and its research. Nonetheless, we hope UCSF's intrinsic grit, accumulated cultural capital, institutional creativity, and capacity for sheer good luck will enable its research mission to meet many of its challenges, internal and external.

Late-breaking news

As this book was going to press, we learned of several developments at UCSF that are directly relevant—although in no way motivated by—our then unpublished proposals for future change. Time is limited, so we describe these only briefly:

1. The Chancellor's office is starting to seek dollars for a general endowment (see chapter 10), to be called the Chancellor's Fund for the Future. Although this fund has not yet been widely promoted, it is being discussed with potential donors.

2. UCSF recently instituted a Physician Scientist Scholar Program, which resembles and significantly extends our proposal in chapter 10. The idea originated in the Department of Medicine, but was adopted by the School of Medicine Dean's office. It provides five years of research support, for a total of $1.25M, for one or two outstanding new clinician-scholars each year, in any of the School's departments. Scholars are chosen by a Steering Committee of faculty from multiple departments. Each scholar's department takes responsibility for paying her or his salary.

3. From the outset, the School of Medicine anticipated future changes in the Basic Science Funding, based on experience with each previous version of the Model. Extensive revision of the Model, effective in 2016, has corrected or decreased many, but not all, of the financial deficiencies we pointed out in chapter 8.

4. UCSF is actively taking steps (publicly announced in January, 2016) to address the housing shortage problems that we mention, by expanding housing opportunities in the Mission Bay area for its students and junior faculty.

As is always the case, many additional changes are "in the works" at UCSF, but have not yet ripened enough to merit discussion.

References

Chapter 1

1. 2014 Annual Financial Report Overview, October 21, 2014. Web 29 February 2016, at http://brm.ucsf.edu/sites/brm.ucsf.edu/files/ wysiwyg/1-1_Annual_Financial_Report_Overview_October_2014.pdf .

2. University of California Medical Centers 13/14 Annual Financial Report (2014) http://finreports.universityofcalifornia.edu/index. php?file=med_ctr/13-14/Med-Centers-13-14-report.pdf .

3. Table of revenues, expenses, and changes in net position, UCSF Annual Financial Report (2014). Web 26 June 2015, at http:// controller.ucsf.edu/fin_statements/files/2014CampusRpt.pdf .

4. Council on Governmental Relations, Finances of Research Universities (June 2014) http://www.cogr.edu/ .

5. Dontes, Arnim. Financing the academic mission: how medical schools work. *Association of American Medical Colleges Group on Business Affairs*, 27 January 2015. Webinar. Web. 11 February 2015, at https://www.aamc.org/members/gba/423462/webinarfinanc- ingtheacademicmission-howmedicalschoolswork.html .

6. University of California Financial Schedules, FY2014. Schedule C: Current funds expenditures by department. Web 29 February 2016, at http://www.ucop.edu/financial-accounting/financial-reports/ campus-financial-schedules/13-14/san-francisco-consolidated.pdf .

7. See page 3 of reference 1, above. The professional fees are referred to by the abbreviation PSA.

8. Data in Figures 4 and 5 come from UCSF Financial Reports for the fiscal years represented.

9. Common Fund, 2014 Higher Education Price Index. Web 23 December 2014, at http://media.bizj.us/view/ img/3864291/hepi-2014-full-report-pdf-9-16-14.pdf .

10. Health care spending doubled, as a percentage of GDP (9% to 17.7%), from 1980 to 2011 (Mercatus Center, http://mercatus.org/publication/us-health- care-spending-more-twice-average-developed-countries), while real GDP grew

2.5-fold over the same interval (US Bureau of Economic Analysis, cited here (http://www.multpl.com/us-gdp-inflation-adjusted/table). Consequently, health care spending must have increased ~five-fold, in inflation-corrected dollars.

11. World Bank, Health expenditure, total (% of GDP). Data for 2010-2014. Web 21 December 2014, at http://data.worldbank.org/indicator/SH.XPD.TOTL.ZS .

12. Letter from N. Brostrom, Executive Vice President of Business, University of California (UC), to UC campus administrators, 29 July 2014. Web 29 February 2016, at http://brm.ucsf.edu/sites/brm.ucsf.edu/files/wysi-wyg/1-12_Executive_Vice_President_Bostrom_letter_od_July_2014.pdf .

13. Associate Vice Chancellor—Budget and Resource Management. Overview of UCSF Debt, 8 December 2015. Web 29 February 2016 at http://brm.ucsf.edu/sites/brm.ucsf.edu/files/wysiwyg/1-13_AVC_BRM_Overview_of_UCSF_Debt_extract.pdf .

14. UCSF projected revenue by 2025 may be as high as $8.5B, making an annual debt payment of $233M less than 3% of revenues. By most standards this low percentage would be considered reasonable, but much of that revenue is restricted in various ways, so that funds available to service the debt will be much smaller than $8.5B.

Chapter 2

1. Table of revenues, expenses, and results of operations, UCSF Annual Financial Report (2014). Web 26 June 2015, at http://controller.ucsf.edu/fin_statements/files/2014CampusRpt.pdf .

2. 2014 Annual Financial Report Overview, October 21, 2014. Web 29 February 2016, at http://brm.ucsf.edu/sites/brm.ucsf.edu/files/wysiwyg/1-1_Annual_Financial_Report_Overview_October_2014.pdf .

3. Associate Vice Chancellor for Budget, UCSF, Report on federal and private contracts & grants (2014). Web 29 February 2016, at http://brm.ucsf.edu/sites/brm.ucsf.edu/files/wysiwyg/2-3_AVC_BRM_Report_on_Federal_and_Private_Contracts_and_Grants_2014.pdf .

4. Associate Vice Chancellor for Budget, UCSF. UCSF Sponsored Project Expense and Overhead Recovery (2014). Web 29 February 2016, at http://brm.ucsf.edu/sites/brm.ucsf.edu/files/wysiwyg/2-4_AVC_BRM_UCSF_Sponsored_Project_Expense_and_Overhead_Recovery_2014.pdf .

5. Associate Dean for Finance, UCSF School of Medicine. Dean's operations and program support (2014), January 2015. Web 29 February, at http://brm.ucsf.edu/sites/brm.ucsf.edu/files/wysiwyg/2-5_Assoc_Dean-Finance_UCSF_School_of_Medicine_Deans_Operations_and_Program_Support_2014.pdf .

6. UCSF Annual Financial Schedules (1979). Web 29 February 2016, at http://brm.ucsf.edu/sites/brm.ucsf.edu/files/wysiwyg/2-6_UCSF_Annual_Financial_Schedules_1979.pdf .

7. Common Fund, 2014 Higher Education Price Index. Web 23 December 2014, at http://media.bizj.us/view/img/3864291/hepi-2014-full-report-pdf-9-16-14.pdf .

8. University of California Office of the President, FY 2015-16 Budget for Current Operations. Web 29 February 2016, at http://ucop.edu/operating-budget/_files/rbudget/2015-16budgetforcurrentoperations_.pdf

9. Associate Vice Chancellor for Budget, UCSF. FY 2014 Patent Allocation Distribution Summary, February 2015. Web 29 February 2016, at http://brm.ucsf.edu/sites/brm.ucsf.edu/files/wysiwyg/2-9_AVC_BRM_UCSF_Patent_Allocation_Summary_2014.pdf .

10. Based on the experience of Eric Vermillion, a former Vice Chancellor for Finance, UCSF, who managed UCSF's Capital Budget process from 1991 to 2013. Details can be found at http://www.ucop.edu/capital-planning/_files/capital/201424/2014-24-capital-financial-plan.pdf and, for reports of prior years, at http://www.ucop.edu/capital-planning/resources/state-capital-improvement-program.html .

11. For instance, compare UCSF's number of students in FY2014 *vs.* that year's enrollment at UC San Diego. The UCSF enrollment is from the Table of primary curriculum enrollment, UCSF Annual Financial Report (2014). Web 26 June 2015, at http://controller.ucsf.edu/fin_statements/files/2014CampusRpt.pdf . Enrollment at UC San Diego is in University of California Annual Financial Report (2014). Web 23 April 2015, at http://finreports.universityof-california.edu/index.php?file=med_ctr/13-14/Med-Centers-13-14-report.pdf.

12. Associate Vice Chancellor—Budget and Resource Management, UCSF. Mission Bay Capital Funding Plan: Source of Funds. Web 29 February 2016, at http://brm.ucsf.edu/sites/brm.ucsf.edu/files/wysiwyg/4-6_AVC_BRM_UCSF_Mission_Bay_Capital_Funding_Plan.pdf . In addition, see two letters from UC Vice President Larry Hershman, University of California Office of the President to UCSF Vice Chancellor Spaulding, on 23 October 2003 (Web 29 February 2016, at http://brm.ucsf.edu/sites/brm.ucsf.edu/files/wysiwyg/2-12b_AVC_BRM_UCSF_Mission_Bay_Funding_Plan_letter_from_UC_VP_Hershman_to_UCSF_VC_Spaulding_October2003.pdf) and 3 December 1999 (Web 29 February 2016, at http://brm.ucsf.edu/sites/brm.ucsf.edu/files/wysiwyg/2-12a_AVC_BRM_Mission_Bay_Capital_Funding_Plan_letter_from_UC_VP_Hershman_to_UCSF_VC_Spaulding_December_1999.pdf .

13. Associate Vice Chancellor for Budget, UCSF. 2014 Report on Utilization of

State Educational Appropriation, 28 May 2015, Web 29 February 2016, at http://brm.ucsf.edu/sites/brm.ucsf.edu/files/wysiwyg/2-13_AVC_BRM_ Report_on_Utilization_of_State_Educational_Appropriation_FY2014.pdf .

14. UCSF Foundation, Financial Report (2014). Web 28 May 2015 at http:// controller.ucsf.edu/fin_statements/files/2014FoundationRpt.pdf .

15. University of California Office of the President, Research policy analysis and coordination, Chapter 9-5000: Distinguishing between private gifts and grants for research. Web 23 April 2015, at http:// ucop.edu/research-policy-analysis-coordination/resources-tools/ contract-and-grant-manual/chapter9/chapter-9-500.html#9-510 .

16. Associate Vice Chancellor for Budget. UCSF Regents Endowment Report for FY 2014, August 2014. Web 29 February 2016, at http://brm.ucsf.edu/ sites/brm.ucsf.edu/files/wysiwyg/2-16a_AVC_BRM_Regents_Endowment_Report_2014.pdf , and UCSF Foundation Endowment Report for FY 2014, dated 30 June 2014 (web 29 February 2016, at http:// brm.ucsf.edu/sites/brm.ucsf.edu/files/wysiwyg/2-16b_AVC_ BRM_UCSF_Foundation_Endowment_Report_2014.pdf .

17. Associate Vice Chancellor for Budget, Report of Regents and Foundation Endowments for UCSF: Medicine Dean and Chancellor Office's extract, July 21, 2015. Web 29 February 2016, at http://brm.ucsf.edu/sites/ brm.ucsf.edu/files/wysiwyg/2-17a_AVC_BRM_Report_on_Regents_ and_Foundation_Endowments-Chancellor_extract_2014.pdf .

18. Vice Chancellor for Development, UCSF. The Infrastructure and Operations Fund, May 2014 and Infrastructure and Operations Fund Q & A, May 27, 2014. Web 29 February 2016, at http://brm.ucsf.edu/ sites/brm.ucsf.edu/files/wysiwyg/2-18a_Vice_Chancellor_-_Development_UCSF_The_Infrastructure_and_Operations_Fund_May2014.pdf .

19. The New FFE is called "Discovery Funds I and II." For more details, see L Kurtzmann, Michael Moritz, Harriet Heyman form UC's largest endowed program for PhD students, UCSF News. Web 23 April 2015, at [http://www.ucsf.edu/news/2013/09/109031/silicon-valley-investor-michael-moritz-and-harriet-heyman-form-largest-endowed.

20. Associate Vice Chancellor for Budget, UCSF. Report on TRIP/STIP Earnings and Equity Payout, FY 2014. Web 29 February 2016, at http:// brm.ucsf.edu/sites/brm.ucsf.edu/files/wysiwyg/2-20_AVC_BRM_ Report_on_TRIP_STIP_Earnings_and_Equity_Payout_2014.pdf .

21. Vice Chancellor for Development, UCSF. Report on donor Profile by Gift Size, (2014), 28 May 2015. Web 29 February 2016, at http:// brm.ucsf.edu/sites/brm.ucsf.edu/files/wysiwyg/2-21_VC_Development_UCSF_Report_on_Donor_Profile_by_Gift_Size.pdf .

Chapter 3

1. UCSF Annual Financial Report (2014). http://controller.ucsf. edu/fin_statements/files/2014CampusRpt.pdf .

2. Interview with Wallace Chan, former national Director of the DHHS Directorate of Cost Accounting, by Eric Vermillion, UCSF Vice Chancellor – Finance, January and February, 2013.

3. Associate Vice Chancellor – Budget, UCSF; 30-year table on UCSF total ICR recovered versus UCSF ICR retained by University of California Office of the President. May, 2015; Web 29 February 2016, at http:// brm.ucsf.edu/sites/brm.ucsf.edu/files/wysiwyg/3-3_AVC_BRM_30_ Year_Table-UCSF_ICR_Retained_by_UC_President_Office.pdf .

4. Resemblance of the M-UP to the Heisenberg Uncertainty Principle is only partly bogus. We challenge readers to identify and quantitate the bogus portion—which, of course, is also subject to the M-UP.

5. Associate Vice Chancellor for Budget, UCSF. UCSF Sponsored Project Expense and Overhead Recovery (2014). Web 29 February 2016, at http://brm. ucsf.edu/sites/brm.ucsf.edu/files/wysiwyg/2-4_AVC_BRM_UCSF_Spon- sored_Project_Expense_and_Overhead_Recovery_2014.pdf .

6. F&A cost pools include, but are not limited to, expenses of the types listed here. Administrative pools include: university/school/college/department/sponsored project administration; accounting and payroll, information technology and computing, human subjects review boards, risk management, affirmative action monitoring, purchasing, communications, and student services. Facilities pools: power and lighting, custodial, facility maintenance and repairs, facilities manage- ment, building depreciation, transportation services, equipment depreciation, capital bond interest, environmental health and safety, security, libraries.

7. UCSF FY 2009-10 Facilities and Administrative Rate Proposal. Diagram created by Eric Vermillion with assistance from Nilo Mia, UCSF Director of Costing Policy, March 2015.

8. W Celis, Navy settles a fraud case on Stanford research costs. *New York Times*, 19 October 1994. Web 10 February 2015, at http:// www.nytimes.com/1994/10/19/us/navy-settles-a-fraud- case-on-stanford-research-costs.html .

9. Associate Vice Chancellor – Controller, UCSF; list of unallowable costs on federal research funds. Web at two locations http://controller.ucsf.edu/pam/files/ CAS_Appendix_A.pdf and http://ucop.edu/research-policy-analysis-coordina- tion/resources-tools/contract-and-grant-manual/chapter7/chapter-7-200.html .

10. H Ledford, Indirect costs: keeping the lights on. *Nature* 514:326-9,

19 November 2014. Web 10 February 2015, at http://www.nature.
com/news/indirect-costs-keeping-the-lights-on-1.16376 .

11. Associate Vice Chancellor – Budget, UCSF, Graph of Indirect cost
    OR rates 1982-2014 based on Federal A-88 agreements. Web 29
    February 2016, at http://brm.ucsf.edu/sites/brm.ucsf.edu/files/wysi-
    wyg/3-11_AVC_BRM_UCSF_Table_of_ICR_OR_Rates_1982-2014.pdf .

12. Associate Vice Chancellor – Budget, UCSF. Graph of ICR Recovery 1982-2014.
    Web 29 February 2016, at http://brm.ucsf.edu/sites/brm.ucsf.edu/files/
    wysiwyg/3-12_AVC_BRM_UCSF_Chart_of_ICR_Recovered_1982-2014.pdf .

13. Associate Vice Chancellor Budget, UCSF. Table of Unrecovered ICR (based
    on 2012 Federal A-88 Agreement, dated May 23, 2012. Web 29 February
    2016, at http://brm.ucsf.edu/sites/brm.ucsf.edu/files/wysiwyg/3-13_AVC_
    BRM_Table_of_Unrecovered_ICR_Based_on_2012_A-88_Agreement.pdf .

14. Few solid facts can be found in the voluminous literature on the administrative
    burdens of federal regulations impose on academic researchers. For useful
    examples in this literature, see a survey of faculty members' perceptions
    of administrative workload (SL Scheider, KK Ness, S Rockwell, K Shaver,
    R Brutkiewicz, 2012 Faculty Workload Survey. Federal Demonstration
    Partnership, Research Report released April 2014. Web 10 April 2015,
    at http://sites.nationalacademies.org/cs/groups/pgasite/documents/
    webpage/pga_087667.pdf) and a National Science Board report recom-
    mending ways to reduce this burden (National Science Board, Task Force on
    Administrative Burdens, Reducing Investigators' Administrative Workload
    for Federally Funded Research. National Science Foundation, March
    10, 2014. http://www.nsf.gov/pubs/2014/nsb1418/nsb1418.pdf).

15. SC Johnston, S Desmond-Hellmann, S Hauser, E Vermillion, N Mia, Predictors
    of negotiated NIH indirect rates at US institutions. *PLoS ONE* 10.1371/
    journal.pone.0121273, pub 20 March 2015. Web 3 April 2015 at http://
    journals.plos.org/plosone/article?id=10.1371/journal.pone.0121273 .

16. This was a 2012 agreement between Wallace Chan, Direc-
    tor of Cost Accounting Administration, DHHS, and then
    UCSF Vice Chancellor of Finance Eric Vermillion.

17. UCSF reviews this rate when it re-negotiates its federal rates and sets it based
    on market experience. The rate in FY 2014 was set in 2012 by then UCSF
    Vice Chancellor of Finance Eric Vermillion, as noted in reference *16*.

18. Nominal NIH budgets in those two years were $23.1B and $30.1B, respectively;
    in 2003 dollars (see *19*, below), the 2014 figure would be $21.3B, which is 78.5%
    of the nominal 2003 NIH budget—that is, less by 21.5%. NIH appropriations
    are listed in NIH History of Congressional Appropriations, Fiscal Years 2000-

2014. Web 10 April 2015 at http://officeofbudget.od.nih.gov/pdfs/FY16/Approp%20%20History%20by%20IC%20through%20FY%202014.pdf .

19. Biomedical Research and Development Price Index, 1950-present. Web 10 April 2015 at http://officeofbudget.od.nih.gov/pdfs/FY16/BRDPI_Values_for_2014_2020.pdf .

20. As shown in Tables 3-2 and 3-3, in FY2014 unrecovered indirect costs on federally- or non-federally funded research were, respectively, 16 cents per TDC dollar (= $82/507) or 29 cents per TDC dollar ($82/288). The difference (= 29-16) is 13 cents.

21. C Kerr, *The Uses of the University*. Cambridge MA, Harvard Univ Press, 1963. It is certainly true that US universities supported significant research in the first half of the 20th century, but in relative terms their research efforts grew much larger after World War II.

22. B Alberts, Overbuilding research capacity. *Science* 329:1257, 2010. Web 6 April 2015, at http://www.sciencemag.org/content/329/5997/1257.full?sid=a0a48272-a1ea-4f4a-b8df-8116af52394f .

Chapter 4

1. Assignable square feet leaves out hallways and utility space that cannot be used academic or clinical purposes. The definition of *asf devoted to research* also specifically excludes space that is *not* used for research—i.e., space devoted primarily to clinical care, teaching, etc.

2. Associate Vice Chancellor—Budget and Resource Management. Summary of UCSF Space Utilization, December 2015. Web 29 February 2016, at http://brm.ucsf.edu/sites/brm.ucsf.edu/files/wysiwyg/4-2_AVC_BRM_Summary_of_UCSF_Space_December_2015.pdf .

3. Executive Vice Chancellor and Provost, UCSF. Campus Administrative Policies: Space Governance and Principles. Policy No. 600-24. 2013. Web October 30, 2015, at http://policies.ucsf.edu/policy/600-24 .

4. Email to one of the authors, October 31, 2015, from Daniel Lowenstein, Executive Vice Chancellor and Provost, UCSF.

5. The following brief history is based on the experience of Eric Vermillion, who joined UCSF's planning and budget staff in 1979 and rose to serve as Associate Vice Chancellor for Budget and Finance in 2003, and as Vice Chancellor for Finance (2010-13).

6. Associate Vice Chancellor—Budget and Resource Management, UCSF. Mission Bay Capital Funding Plan: Source of Funds. Web 29 February 2016, at http://brm.ucsf.edu/sites/brm.ucsf.edu/files/wysiwyg/4-6_AVC_

BRM_UCSF_MissionBay_Capital_Funding_Plan.pdf . The data is from the latest update of this plan, dated February 25, 2016. Tables 4-3 and 4-4 include only data from parts of the plan whose status was complete on that date, and thus omit all "pending" or "programming" items.

7. See chapter 2 and reference *13* of that chapter.

8. State funds in 2009 paid for a $35M capital improvement for Telemedicine and PRIME-US Education Facilities (see Telemedicine project funding authorization. Web 29 February 2016, at http://brm.ucsf.edu/sites/brm.ucsf.edu/files/wysiwyg/4-8_UCSF_Telemedicine_Project_Funding_Authorization.pdf). In 2015, UCSF received the first payment (of a total that will come to $21.7M) from UC for seismic retrofit and renovation of the Clinical Sciences Building on the Parnassus Campus (see AB 94 info CSB project 2015.pdf (Web 1 March 2016, at http://brm.ucsf.edu/sites/brm.ucsf.edu/files/wysiwyg/4-8_AB_94_UCSF_CSB_project_funding_authorization.pdf). Funds for both these projects were paid from State Bonds for UC.

9. Associate Vice Chancellor—Budget and Resource Management, UCSF. Overview of UCSF Debt. December 8, 2015. Web 29 February 2016, at http://brm.ucsf.edu/sites/brm.ucsf.edu/files/wysiwyg/4-9_AVC_BRM_Overview_of_UCSF_Debt_extract_December2015.pdf .

10. UCSF. Long Range Development Plan (LRDP). Web 8 November 2015 at http://www.ucsf.edu/about/cgr/current-projects/lrdp .

11. B Alberts, Overbuilding research capacity. *Science* 329:1257, 2010. Web 6 April 2015, at http://www.sciencemag.org/content/329/5997/1257.full?sid=a0a48272-a1ea-4f4a-b8df-8116af52394f . We also cited Alberts's editorial in chapter 3.

12. UCSF A-88 agreement with DHHS (Division of Cost Allocation), Exhibit A, page 1, Organized Research on-campus cost components {July 2013-June 2104), dated May 23, 2102. Web 29 February 2016, at http://brm.ucsf.edu/sites/brm.ucsf.edu/files/wysiwyg/4-12_AVC_BRM_UCSF_A88_Agreement_Exhibit_A_page_1.pdf .

13. During this period, one of the authors, Eric Vermillion, was responsible for the financial analysis UCSF used in deciding whether to build such facilities. See reference *5*, above.

14. California state legislator John Garamendi sponsored the bill, which is Section 15820.21 of the California Government Code.

15. One might wonder why the University of California would need to have a law passed to be able to use its own revenue. The reason is based on a long standing agreement between the University and the State that UC would use a portion of its ICR to subvent (or in a sense, pay back) the State educational appropriation,

based on a negotiated formula. Once an agreement becomes part of the State Budget Act, it becomes law and therefore requires a new law to change it.

Chapter 5

1. Interim Senior Vice Chancellor, Finance and Administration, UCSF. UCSF Financial Plan. October 27, 2015. Web 29 February 2016, at http://brm.ucsf.edu/sites/brm.ucsf.edu/files/wysiwyg/5-1_Interim_ SVC_FandA_UCSF_Financial_Plan_Fall_October2015.pdf .

2. Associate Vice Chancellor, Finance, UCSF. Mission Bay Capital Funding Plan: Source of Funds. Web 29 February 2016, at http://brm.ucsf. edu/sites/brm.ucsf.edu/files/wysiwyg/5-2_AVC_BRM_UCSF_Mission_Bay_Capital_Funding_Plan.pdf . See also Fig. 4-3, above.

3. Joint committee meeting on grounds and buildings, UC Regents meeting, September 16, 2010. Amendment to the UCSF capital improvement budget for new UCSF medical center facility at Mission Bay. Web 13 January 2016, at http://regents.universityofcalifornia.edu/minutes/2010/joint9.pdf .

4. UCSF Long Range Development Plan. November 2014. Web 29 February 2016, at https://www.ucsf.edu/cgr/cgr-projects/lrdp .

5. UCSF Annual Financial Schedules (1979). Web 29 February 2016, at http://brm.ucsf.edu/sites/brm.ucsf.edu/files/ wysiwyg/2-6_UCSF_Annual_Financial_Schedules_1979.pdf .

6. Email to Eric Vermillion on January 14, 2016 from Debora Obley, Associate Vice President, Budget Analysis and Planning, University of California, Office of the President (UCOP). Getting the data for FY 1971 required a search through paper records in the UCOP library.

7. As recalled by Eric Vermillion, then a member of the UCSF Chancellor's Budget & Planning staff, and subsequently UCSF Vice Chancellor Finance.

8. A subvention, a term of art in governmental operations, occurs when one government entity "grants" funds to another in support of a specific purpose. While the term does not always imply deception, this use of ICR to subvent the SEA did manage to deceive some faculty and officials, although understanding how it did so requires close attention. Because the state of California wanted UC to use some of the (then) new ICR to offset its costs in supporting the University, a formulaic way to accomplish this was devised in the 1960s. Even today, UC continues to "subvent" the State General Funds appropriation with what it terms "UC General Funds," which include ICR. For decades, such subvented funds were contained within the amount of the State budget each campus received (i.e., what UCSF calls the SEA), allocated by the UC Presidents

Office. Unaware that some of their own ICR was included in the total, most UC staff and faculty thought that all the money in their allocated portion of "State General Funds" (known as "19900 funds," in Campus parlance) came from the state, but that was not the case. Only in the past five years or so, when the great recession put extreme stress on UC funding and the state cut almost a billion dollars from the UC budget, did UC uncouple its UC General Funds from the State General Funds, so that campuses could keep all their earned ICR revenues. While each campus is still required to contribute a dollar amount of its own revenues as a share of the state subvention, now campuses can choose what color of money they use for the subvention.

9. As UCSF preferred, the formula allocated ~20% of each year's ICR to each campus, in proportion to the ICR it earned. But the remaining ~80% was split, of which slightly more than half went to the UC General Fund (to subvent state funds; see reference *10*, above), while the rest was allocated to campuses according to criteria—for instance, numbers of undergraduate students per campus—quite unrelated to either research or ICR.

10. For the 27.7% rate, see Associate Vice Chancellor–Budget & Resource Management. UCSF History of Federal Negotiated F&A Rates–Organized Research. Web 29 February 2016, at http://brm.ucsf.edu/follow-money-financing-research-ucsf-references . For current rates at a range of research universities, see SC Johnston, S Desmond-Hellmann, S Hauser, E Vermillion, N Mia, Predictors of negotiated NIH indirect rates at US institutions. *PLoS ONE* 10.1371/journal.pone.0121273, pub 20 March 2015. Web 3 April 2015 at http://journals.plos.org/plosone/article?id=10.1371/journal.pone.0121273 .

11. Campus Core funds currently include ICR, the SEA, investment income, tuition and fees, and income from auxiliaries such as housing, parking and recreation, plus patent income and some endowment income, gifts and certain internal assessments.

12. For the change in state funding between 1991 and 1995, see UCSF Annual Financial Reports for those years. With respect to the regulatory changes that affected what the university could charge as direct costs, note that these changes were not described in Chapter 3, which focused instead on indirect costs.

13. One of the authors (HRB) vividly remembers this occasion.

14. A major assumption in operational planning for the Mission Bay research campus was that state funds would provide an annual allocation of ~$14M (that is, $14 per square foot times approximately a million asf), to help defray costs of maintenance, utilities, and operations costs for eligible facilities. Longstanding agreements obligated the state to fund a share of the operations, maintenance and utility costs of UC buildings determined "eligible" for state

support, including teaching facilities, support facilities and research facilities. As economic problems persisted through the 1990s and the 2000s, however, the State (and the UC President's office, which sets funding priorities for all UC) increasingly backed away from many funding commitments. So, in this case, and with the state's agreement, only teaching-related facilities (needed for UC's increased enrollment of undergraduate students) would receive either capital funds or operations, maintenance and utility funds during these years. Funds for new research facilities have not been reinstated. A few exceptions in UCSF's favor should be noted: (i) state funds were provided for a small portion of the Genentech Hall building at Mission Bay, based on a long standing agreement to fund replacement space for an older building at Parnassus; (ii) state funds for maintenance and utilities were also provided for a portion of the QB3 building (Byers Hall), because it was built at the State's insistence under the earlier California Institutes for Science and Innovation Initiative. Even for these buildings, the state provided only ~50% of capital, maintenance, and utility funds—thus further underlining the state's lack of reliability as a financial partner.

15. The firm, Kaufmann-Hall, was nationally known for developing financial modeling tools for medical centers, but had not previously produced models that incorporated the financial eccentricities of a university engaged in teaching and research, with accounting rules different from those required of medical centers. The silo-based models were driven by federal regulations requiring different sets of books for hospitals and universities.

16. Vice Chancellor–Finance, UCSF. Report on Operational Excellence and Departmental Budget Savings, August 1, 2013. Web 29 February 2016, at http://brm.ucsf.edu/sites/brm.ucsf.edu/files/wysiwyg/5-16_VC_Finance_UCSF_Report_on_Operational_Excellence_and_Budget_Savings_August_2013.pdf .

17. The EBC's membership has remained constant, but principal financial officers of each Control Point have joined the group as an ex-officio associates, allowing both principal Control Point officers and their financial right hands to participate in EBC discussions. This change led later to formation of a committee (now called the Budget and Investment Working Group), composed of Control Point financial officers, their seconds, and the Chancellor's Budget and Resource Management staff. The latter group hashes out nitty-gritty details of problems, proposals, technical solutions, and implementation mechanisms, along with more detailed discussion of details of financial reports.

18. Interim Senior Vice Chancellor, Finance and Administration, UCSF Financial Plan *Fall* 2015, Oct 13, 2015. Web 29 February 2061, at http://brm.ucsf.edu/sites/brm.ucsf.edu/files/wysiwyg/5-18_Interim_SVC_FandA_UCSF_Financial_Plan_Fall_October_2015.pdf . The final Annual

Financial Report may not be available before this book goes to press.

19. For instance, a budget bill signed into law on 18 December 2015 gives the NIH a 6% increase in funds for 2016, relative to 2015. But this, the first substantial raise in more than a decade, does not quite recoup losses in constant NIH dollars since 2003, and the "deal struck in October by legislators and [President] Obama provides almost no room for further boosts in 2017." S Reardon, C Cesar, H Lebford. US biomedicine nets budget win. Nature 528: 446 (2015).

Chapter 6

1. Associate Vice Chancellor—Budget and Resource Management, UCSF. 2014 Annual Financial Report Overview, October 21, 2014. Web 29 February 2016, at http://brm.ucsf.edu/sites/brm.ucsf.edu/files/wysiwyg/1-1_Annual_Financial_Report_Overview_October_2014.pdf . Instead of citing the subsequently published official Financial Report for that year (which we have cited in multiple previous chapters—for instance, reference 3 in chapter 1), we cite the overview, which contains headcount information, which is correct but not included in the later version.

2. The UC retirement system had been more than 100% funded for several decades, and for two decades the plan had received no employee or employer contributions. As a consequence of the 2001-04 "dot.com" recession, followed by the 2008 'great' recession, the UC system was forced to begin requiring both types of contributions again, because the retirement system's projected funds fell into the 80% funded range, and UC policy requires that it be 100% funded.

3. S. Marshall et al., Academic Affairs, UCSF, An Insider's Guide to advancement and promotion at UCSF. October 23, 2008. Web 23 December 2014 at http://academicaffairs.ucsf.edu/ccfl/media/Events/fdd2011/advancement_and_promotion_Oct_08_slides.pdf .

4. Associate Vice Chancellor—Budget and Resource Management, UCSF. Faculty Salary Fund Source Profile, April, 2015. Web 1 March 2016, at http://brm.ucsf.edu/sites/brm.ucsf.edu/files/wysiwyg/6-4_AVC_BRM_UCSF_Faculty_Salary_Fund_Source_Profile_FY2014_0.pdf . This file contains the salary and faculty profile data for FY2014, derived from faculty salary ledgers, that is included in Tables 6-2, 6-3, and 6-4, as well as Figures 6-1, 6-2, and 6-3. It should be noted, however, that ~150 "faculty" (who were not explicitly recorded as belonging to one of the five~ series described in the text) are not included in data reported in those tables. Defined as belonging to a specified faculty series, the faculty headcount was 2,395, and their total salaries amounted to $492M. Both figures are less than those reported in the UCSF

Annual Financial Report for that year (reference *1*, above), which put the headcount at 2,545 and total faculty salary at \$542M (Table 6-1 and reference *1*). The latter numbers are greater—by, respectively, 150 people (6.3%) and \$40M (10.2%)—than we found by defining faculty by their assignment to a faculty series. Possible reasons for this discrepancy include: (i) faculty who did belong to a specific series may have been mistakenly unlabeled as such in the financial records surveyed for Tables 6-2 to 6-4; alternatively, (ii) some of the difference may represent individuals who are in fact "academic non-faculty" (a large category, defined in the legend of Table 6-1) but were incorrectly designated as faculty in reference *1*. Fortunately, the discrepancies are not large enough to call into question any inferences we draw from the data.

5. S.A. Bunton and R.A. Sloane, The redistribution of tenure tracks for U.S. medical school faculty: clinical MED faculty. Association of American Medical Colleges, *Analysis in Brief* 15(5) (2015). Web pdf 21 May 2015 at https://www.aamc.org/download/432328/data/may2015redis-tributionofrenureracksusmedicalschoolfacultypart1.pdf .

6. S.A. Bunton, The relationship between tenure and guaranteed salary for U.S. medical school faculty. Association of American Medical Colleges, *Analysis in Brief*, 9(6) (2010).

7. Report of UCSF In-residence Task Force, 19 February 1999. Web 2 December 2015, at http://academicaffairs.ucsf.edu/academic-personnel/media/inresidencereport2005.pdf .

8. In this chapter, "department types" fall into four categories: academic clinical departments; academic basic science departments; organized research units (ORUs); and "other." Both types of academic department are represented in UCSF's four different schools. The largest category includes 26 "clinical" departments, each named for a clinical specialty (e.g., Otolaryngology, Family Health Care Nursing); this category includes three units in the School of Dentistry, 20 in the School of Medicine, two in the School of Nursing, and one in the School of Pharmacy. The 12 "basic science" departments include one in the School of Dentistry (Cell and Tissue Biology), seven in the School of Medicine (Anatomy; Anthropology, History, and Social Medicine; Biochemistry and Biophysics; Cellular and Molecular Pharmacology; Epidemiology and Biostatistics; Microbiology and Immunology; Physiology), two in the School of Nursing (Physiological Nursing, Social and Behavioral Sciences); and two in the School of Pharmacy (Bioengineering and Therapeutic Sciences, Pharmaceutical Chemistry). UCSF's seven ORUs include the Proctor Foundation, Cardiovascular Research Institute, the Diabetes Center, the Helen Diller Family Comprehensive Cancer Center, the Institute of Neurodegenerative

Disease, the Institute for Health and Aging, and the Philip R. Lee Institute for Health Policies. The "other" category includes two units: Dean's Office of the School of Medicine; Osher Center of Integrative Medicine.

9. Data for these increases pertain to the School of Medicine only, and are cited in chapter 7.

10. The source of this data is the document cited in reference 4 to this chapter.

11. Association of American Medical Colleges, Sponsored program salary support to medical school faculty in 2009. January, 2011. Web 13 January 2015 https://www.aamc.org/download/170836/data/aibvol11_no1.pdf .

Chapter 7

1. HR Bourne. *Paths to Innovation: Discovering recombinant DNA, oncogenes, and prions, in one medical school, over one decade.* University of California Medical Humanities Consortium and University of California Press, Berkeley, CA, 2011.

2. Herbert Evans, a renowned physiologist, made this remark in the mid-1960s to LH Smith, Jr, then chairman of UCSF's Department of Medicine. Quoted in reference *1*, above, p 2.

3. The dean was William Reinhardt. The CVRI director was Julius H Comroe, Jr, who instigated the successful coup to unseat the Chancellor, as described in chapter 2 of reference *1*, above.

4. ORU faculty typically hold joint appointments in regular academic departments and may teach in those departments and even assume limited clinical responsibilities, when appropriate; nonetheless, the ORU usually takes primary responsibility for their promotions, their laboratories, and administration of their research grants and contracts.

5. See C Kerr, *A UC President's View of the Expanding Research Community.* Interviewer: Nancy M Rockafellar, The UCSF Oral History Program, Kalmanoviz Library, UCSF, San Francisco. Interviews December 19,1994, El Cerrito, CA.

6. For the data, see NIH research grants, 1952-1985, a graph on p 65 of reference *1*.

7. Except for the CVRI, which Comroe organized a decade or so earlier, non-clinical research at UCSF was rather old-fashioned before Rutter came. See reference *1*.

8. The discoveries are described in reference *1*. Herbert Boyer, then in UCSF's Department of Microbiology, discovered how to cut, splice, and recombine genes and DNA fragments into the bacterial genome, in collaboration with Stanley Cohen, Stanford University. Boyer later co-founded Genentech, the biotechnology company, in collaboration with Robert Swanson. Michael Bishop and Harold Varmus, also in Microbiology, discovered *src*, the first oncogene. Stanley Prusiner, in Neurology, discovered

prions and their role in transmission of Creuzfeldt-Jakob disease.

9. Information about UCSF's contributions and discoveries (Table 7-1) and scientific awards and prizes received by UCSF faculty (Table 7-2) came from multiple sources, including: reference *1* in the present chapter; the authors' conversations with UCSF researchers; a web survey by the authors, looking for outstanding accomplishments by UCSF personnel; and helpful suggestions from Kristen Bole, UCSF University Relations.

10. Names of these departments, their classification as clinical *vs.* non-clinical/ basic, and the schools to which they belong are listed in chapter 6, reference 7. Note that the 12 non-clinical departments, although broadly classified as "basic science departments," include four whose research focuses on social science; of these, two are in the School of Medicine and two in the School of Nursing.

11. Associate Vice Chancellor for Budget, UCSF. UCSF Sponsored Project Expense and Overhead Recovery (2014). Web 29 February 2016, at http://brm.ucsf. edu/sites/brm.ucsf.edu/files/wysiwyg/7-11_AVC_BRM_UCSF_Spon-sored_Project_Expense_and_Overhead_Recovery_2014.pdf .

12. Associate Vice Chancellor – Budget & Resource Management; UCSF ICR Benchmarking Data Report for FY 2013-14. Web 29 February, at http://brm.ucsf.edu/sites/brm.ucsf.edu/files/wysi-wyg/7-13_AVC_BRM_UCSF_ICR_Benchmarking_Data_FY13-14.pdf .

13. This M-UP requires some kind of ruler to compare the values of different kinds of square feet: dry-lab *vs.* wet-lab *vs.* clinical-lab *vs.* whatever-lab. What kind of value do we mean? Is the correct measure something like indirect costs recovered per square foot, a kind of "landlord's rule"? Instead, should we base its value on how much space of each particular flavor the present research population covets? On the relative value to science or humanity of various kinds of research?

14. Common Fund, 2014 Higher Education Price Index. Web 23 December 2014, at http://media.bizj.us/view/img/3864291/hepi-2014-full-report-pdf-9-16-14. pdf . Note also: (i) over the period in question, this price index shows virtually the same percentage change in prices as does the Biomedical Research and Development Price Index, which focuses entirely on research expenditures; (ii) comparisons in this chapter do not include dollars that came to UCSF as a result of the American Recovery and Reinvestment Act of 2009 (ARRA).

15. Associate Vice Chancellor for Budget, UCSF. UCSF Sponsored Project Expense and Overhead Recovery (2004). Web 29 February 2016, at http://brm.ucsf. edu/sites/brm.ucsf.edu/files/wysiwyg/7-16_AVC_BRM_UCSF_Spon-sored_Project_Expense_and_Overhead_recovery_2004.pdf .

16. Dollar data in this and the following paragraphs are from references *11* and *14*.

Chapter 8

1. S. Masters, Associate Dean for Curriculum, School of Medicine, UCSF, in a telephone interview September 8, 2015.

2. K Hopkins. SARS, malaria, and the microarray. *TheScientist*, November 21 2005. Web 15 July 2015 at http://www.the-scientist.com/?articles.view/articleNo/16860/title/SARS--Malaria--and-the-Microarray/ .

3. See publications listed in David Julius, UCSF Profiles, at http://profiles.ucsf.edu/david.julius .

4. See publications listed in Nirao Shah, UCSF Profiles, at http://profiles.ucsf.edu/nirao.shah .

5. N Zeliadt. Profile of Kevan M Shokat, *Proc Nat Acad Sci USA* 108:15046-52 (2012). Web 15 July 2015 at http://www.pnas.org/content/109/28/11057.full .

6. See publications listed in Ronald Vale, UCSF Profiles, at http://profiles.ucsf.edu/ron.vale .

7. Lasker Award Winner Peter Walter, *Nature Medicine* 20:1112-4, 2014. Web 15 July 2015 http://www.nature.com/nm/journal/v20/n10/full/nm.3683.html.

8. J Fleischman. The ribosome profiler, Jonathan Weissman. *ASCB Post*, July 6 2015. Web 15 July 2015 at http://ascb.org/the-ribosomal-profiler-jonathan-weissman/ .

9. Interview with J Weissman in his Mission Bay office, 17 April 2015.

10. Associate Vice Chancellor for Budget, UCSF. UCSF Sponsored Project Expense and Overhead Recovery (2014). Web 29 February 2016, at http://brm.ucsf.edu/sites/brm.ucsf.edu/files/wysiwyg/2-4_AVC_BRM_UCSF_Sponsored_Project_Expense_and_Overhead_Recovery_2014.pdf .

11. Personal communication from C. Desjarlais, assistant dean of UCSF Graduate Division, June 2015.

12. Associate Vice Chancellor – Budget & Resource Management. UCSF ICR Benchmarking Data Report for FY 2013-14. July 2 July 2015. Web 29 February 2016, at http://brm.ucsf.edu/sites/brm.ucsf.edu/files/wysiwyg/7-13_AVC_BRM_UCSF_ICR_Benchmarking_Data_FY13-14.pdf .

13. HR Bourne. *Paths to Innovation: Discovering recombinant DNA, oncogenes, and prions, in one medical school, over one decade.* University of California Medical Humanities Consortium and University of California Press, Berkeley, CA, 2011.

14. The HHMI pays salaries and benefits, plus substantial research funds, to the PIs themselves; UCSF receives rent for the space occupied by these faculty members.

15. Associate Vice Chancellor—Budget, UCSF. 2014 Report of HHM investigator space occupancy. Web 29 February 2016, at http://brm.ucsf.edu/sites/brm.ucsf.edu/files/wysiwyg/8-15_AVC_BRM_

UCSF_HHMI_Investigator_occupancy_inventor_2014.pdf .

16. American Association of Medical Colleges, Report on Medical School Faculty salaries, 2013-2014. The AAMC provides online instructions on how to obtain a copy of this survey (Web 2 August 2015, at https://www.aamc.org/download/369956/data/currentgfanowissue.pdf). The authors examined the survey in the Academic Affairs division of the office of UCSF's Dean of the School of Medicine on July 14, 2015.

17. Rent Jungle, Rent trend data in San Francisco, CA, May 2015. Web 29 July 2015, at https://www.rentjungle.com/average-rent-in-san-francisco-rent-trends .

18. NIH. Ruth L Kirschstein National Research Service Award (NRSA) stipends, tuition/fees, and other budgetary levels effective for fiscal year 2015. Web 26 July 2015, at http://grants.nih.gov/grants/guide/notice-files/NOT-OD-14-046.html .

19. Zillow Home Value Index. San Francisco home prices and values, May 31, 2015. Web 29 July 2015, at http://www.zillow.com/san-francisco-ca/home-values/ .

20. Interview with Daniel Lowenstein, UCSF Executive Vice Chancellor, in his office on July 22, 2015.

21. Interview with Joseph Derisi, in his office, on April 3, 2015.

22. W. Benow, Creating operational efficiencies with community engagement. Presentation to a Chief Business Officers meeting at the Association of American Medical Colleges, September 27, 2013. UCSF Chancellor Sam Hawgood gave us a copy of this presentation in early March, 2016.

23. C.L. Leathers, Director, Academic Personnel. ABOG tools of the trade, Presentation May 21, 2009. Web 30 July 2015, at http://academicaffairs.ucsf.edu/academic-personnel/compensation-benefits/downloads/ABOGToolsoftheTrade052209CLL.pdf .

24. University of California Academic Personnel Manual. Web 20 July 2015, at http://www.ucop.edu/academic-personnel-programs/academic-personnel-policy/ .

25. Dean's office, School of Medicine, UCSF. Basic science Departments: Resource allocation model, a presentation to department mangers on August 8, 2014. A. Paardekooper, Interim Vice Dean of the School of Medicine, UCSF, communicated this presentation to the authors on June 3, 2015.

26. For instance, reference 25 explicitly states that: the School of Medicine's Dean's office will absorb annual changes to the SEA; the Dean's office will partner with basic science departments in preparing recruiting packages for new faculty; contributions from the Dean's office to the BSFM will include multiple resources, including the SEA and indirect costs from sponsored projects; if a faculty slot is vacated, the associated BSFM funds

revert temporarily to the Dean's office, to be shared by all departments until the slot is occupied; the Dean and the basic science department chairs, acting as an executive committee, will agree on filling these slots.

27. Specifically, the BSFM would pay ~$100,000 of actual salary (= $130K/1.297). The $181,500 in addition would come to a total salary of $281,500, and the grant would pay the corresponding benefits, for a total of 1.297 x $181,500. The number of basic science faculty with gross salaries greater than $281,500 was determined by surveying 2014 salaries of professor-rank UCSF basic science faculty (see University of California Employee Pay. Web 24 October 2015 at https://ucannualwage.ucop.edu/wage/ . Of the nine individuals whose salaries were greater than $281,500, five were in the School of Medicine and four in the School of Pharmacy.

28. The total faculty salaries assume that professors at each faculty rank earn the median UCSF salary listed in reference *16*, and that their average benefits are 29.7% of total salary. Thus the total salary includes two assistant professors at $118,000 per year x 1.297 (= $304,000), two associate professors at $145,000 x 1.297 (= $374,000), and four professors at $225,000 x 1.297 (=2,322,000). Together, this amounts to $3,000,000 in salaries plus benefits.

29. The departments' share of faculty salaries, based on the presentation to department managers (reference *25*), would include 48% of the total $678,000 for assistant and associate professor salaries, or $324,000 (= 0.48 x $678,000) and $956,000 for 8 associate professors (= 0.41 x 8 x $225,000 x 1.297 for benefits), for a total—if the initial estimates are correct—of $1,280,000. Presumably grants would pay the rest, or $1,720,000.

30. Human Resources assesses payments from departments that are pro-rated in ways that depend on numbers of department personnel and their positions and responsibilities. Similarly, Research Management Services, a central office responsible for pre-award administration of grant applications, pro-rates its charges to the number and type of applications it processes in a given year. Rather than try to calculate fictional amounts, we estimated both figures from conversations with managers of basic science departments.

31. The charge per graduate student at the 2015 rate assessed by UCSF's Integrated Funding Model for graduate programs, which distributes money to graduate programs from departments. We estimate 2.5 students for each of 12 PIs.

32. To pay a host of disparate charges, ranging from pencils, paper, and telephones to staff computers, and many other kinds of charges. This number also is arbitrary, based on conversations with department managers.

33. Arbitrary estimations of salary plus benefits. In real departments these salaries depend on rank and responsibilities of individual staff. See also, Table 8.4.

34. This number is calculated from figures in the BSFM plan for 2015, cited in reference *25*, above. For various faculty ranks, the amounts supplied by the BSFM would be: $150,000 for two assistant professors, at $75,000 each; $170,000 for two associate professors, at $85,000 each; $420,000 for four full professors, at $105,000 each; and $520,000 for four additional full professors, at $130,000 each. (The BSFM offers different amounts for two categories of professors, depending on their "step" at full professor rank; we arbitrarily assigned half of these fictional professors to be in the lower category, half in the upper.) The BSFM's total contribution for faculty salaries, then, would come to $1,260,000. Amounts for staff (12 staff at $50,000 each) and "base" administrative payments ($335,000) are as listed in reference *25*.

35. UCSF Graduate Division, Basic Sciences—Demographics. Web 17 September 2015 at https://graduate.ucsf.edu/basic-sciences-demographics .

36. UCSF figures reflect status of former students, assessed in summer and fall 2012 (UCSF Graduate Division. Basic Sciences—career outcomes. Web 27 July 2015, at https://graduate.ucsf.edu/basic-sciences-career-outcomes). National averages are from National Institutes of Health, Biomedical Research Workforce Working Group Report, June 14, 2012. Web 27 July 2015 at http://acd.od.nih.gov/biomedical_research_wgreport.pdf .

37. The national average is from the Biomedical Research Workforce Working Group Report, as cited in reference *36*, above.

38. The 10 graduate programs in basic sciences include Bioengineering, Biological and Medical Informatics, Biomedical Sciences, Biophysics, Chemistry and Chemical Biology, Developmental and Stem Cell Biology, Neuroscience, Oral and Craniofacial, Pharmaceutical Science and Pharmacogenomics, and Tetrad. (The Tetrad program combines subprograms in Biochemistry and Molecular Biology, Cell Biology, Developmental Biology, and Genetics.) The five social science graduate programs include Epidemiology and Translational, History of Health Sciences, Medical Anthropology, Nursing, and Sociology.

39. The total number of social science graduate students, including the PhD in Nursing program's 94 students, was 165, according to: (i) UCSF Graduate Division, Social Sciences PhD Programs — Demographics. Web 17 September 2015 at https://graduate.ucsf.edu/social-sciences-demographics ; (ii) Graduate Division, Nursing PhD: Demographics. Web 18 September 2015, at https://graduate.ucsf.edu/programs/nursing-phd-demographics .

40. Annual tuition and fees for in-state graduate students are tabulated for FY 2015 by the UCSF Graduate Division (Web 3 August 2015, at http://registrar.ucsf.edu/registration/fees/graddiv). The graduate stipend ($32,500 per year in FY2015) is fixed by agreement of directors of

all 10 basic science graduate programs in January before interviews
with the next years' prospective students, according to David Morgan,
director of the Tetrad program, in an email, August 3, 2015.

41. Average time-to-degree was calculated for 504 students who graduated
between 2002 and 2006. UCSF Graduate Division. Web 26 July 2014,
at http://graduate.ucsf.edu/basic-sciences-aggregate-ttd .

42. The UCSF Graduate Division stressed that these rough percentage estimates are
by no means precise, owing to the large numbers of graduate programs and
separate grants and institutional funds involved. In other words, the estimates
provide unbiased but at best highly approximate numbers. In this regard, it
should be noted that at the national level estimates of biomedical PhD training
costs and relative contributions from the sources that pay them are notoriously
inadequate. While NIH itself pays much of the cost, it has so far not quantified the number of graduate students supported by its research grants, how
many NIH dollars they receive from these grants, or the proportion of these
costs paid by institutions that train graduate students. Moreover, individual
institutions rarely reveal how much they contribute to defray these costs.

43. For discussions of biomedical graduate education and use of the PhD degree
to provide labor for laboratories, see B Alberts, MW Kirschner, S Tilghman,
H Varmus. Rescuing US biomedical research f rom its systemic flaws. *Proc
Natl Acad Sci* 111:5773-7, 2014, and HR Bourne, Is 6 years too long to get
a Ph.D. in biomedical science? *FASEB J* 29:357-360, 2015. The latter paper
also discusses the number of years required for a biomedical PhD degree.

44. The estimated ~$24M spent on about 500 postdocs comes to ~$48,000
per postdoc year. Each student year, as stipulated above, costs about
$50,000, whether it comes out of a PI's grant or from another source,
and thus to the PI is virtually the same as the cost of a postdoc.

Chapter 9

1. Of these fold-differences, the first three are derived from data in Table 7-4; the
fold-difference in sponsored dollars (contracts and grants) is the quotient
of 73% divided by 18% growth (for clinical *vs.* basic science departments,
respectively, both in nominal dollars) from 2004 to 2014, in Fig. 7-1.

2. The examples were collected by polling 18 UCSF leaders and researchers, including seven chairs or division chiefs,
five wet-lab scientists, and six dry-lab scientists.

3. See publications listed in Fahy's and Woodruff's UCSF Profiles. Web 12 August 2015, at http://profiles.ucsf.edu/john.

fahy and http://profiles.ucsf.edu/prescott.woodruff .

4. See publications listed in their UCSF Profiles. Web 12 August 2015, at http://profiles.ucsf.edu/louis.ptacek and http://profiles.ucsf.edu/ying-hui.fu .

5. See publications listed in his UCSF Profile. Web 12 August 2015, at http://profiles.ucsf.edu/stephen.hauser .

6. See publications in his UCSF profile. Web 12 August 2015, at http://profiles.ucsf.edu/david.rowitch .

7. See publications in his UCSF profile. Web 12 August 2015, at http://profiles.ucsf.edu/richard.locksley .

8. See publications listed in their UCSF Profiles. Web 12 August 2015, at http://profiles.ucsf.edu/robert.grant and http://profiles.ucsf.edu/diane.havlir .

9. JC Watts, et al. Transmission of multiple system atrophy prions to transgenic mice. Proc Nat Acad Sci 110:19555-560, 2013. Web August 12 2015, at http://www.pnas.org/content/110/48/19555.full.pdf?sid=f693740d-5f8e-416e-9380-715817f1fa8c .

10. Associate Vice Chancellor for Budget, UCSF. UCSF Sponsored Project Expense and Overhead Recovery (2014). Web 29 February 2016, at http://brm.ucsf.edu/sites/brm.ucsf.edu/files/wysiwyg/2-4_AVC_BRM_UCSF_Sponsored_Project_Expense_and_Overhead_Recovery_2014.pdf .

11. Administrative units are listed in chapter 6, reference 7.

12. For a list of 231 different kinds of NIH grants, see National Institutes of Health. Grants & Funding: Activity codes search results. Web 18 August 2015, at http://grants.nih.gov/grants/funding/ac_search_results.htm.

13. Dr. Hellmann left UCSF in 2014 to become CEO of the Bill and Melinda Gates Foundation, and was replaced as Chancellor by Sam Hawgood. She was not the "research aggregator" just mentioned.

14. UCSF. Research partnerships. Web 18 August 2015 at https://www.ucsf.edu/about/research-partnerships .

15. University of California Financial Schedules, FY2014. Schedule C: Current funds expenditures by department; http://www.ucop.edu/financial-accounting/financial-reports/campus-financial-schedules/13-14/san-francisco-consolidated.pdf .

16. The diagram is based on a personal communication to the authors on June 3, 2015 by A Paardekooper, then the Associate Dean of the UCSF School of Medicine.

17. 2014 Annual Financial Report Overview, October 21, 2014. Web 29 February 2016, at http://brm.ucsf.edu/sites/brm.ucsf.edu/files/wysiwyg/1-1_Annual_Financial_Report_Overview_October_2014.pdf .

18. As described in the main text, above, UCSF defines basic science departments in several ways. Here the definition includes the five School of

Medicine departments whose research focuses on wet-lab biology (i.e., Anatomy, Biochemistry and Biophysics, Cellular and Molecular Pharmacology, Physiology, Microbiology and Immunology), plus Epidemiology and Anthropology, History and Social Medicine. Of these seven, Biochemistry and Biophysics is unusual in that its budget is rarely in arrears.

19. These clinicians' contentions are intensified by the high regard and generosity some of UCSF's former leaders accorded to basic scientists, prosperity of expanding clinical departments and their research, and fiscal constraints imposed by flat-lined NIH budgets and contracted state support for university faculty salaries and research.

20. Bruce Wintroub, interview December 1, 2014. At the time of this interview, in addition to his job as chair of the Department of Dermatology, Wintroub was acting Dean of the School of Medicine.

21. In the Department of Medicine, examples include: cardiology; rheumatology; infectious disease; and pulmonary, critical care, and allergy and immunology.

22. This person preferred not to be named.

23. Robert Nussbaum, interview November 24, 2014. At the time of this interview, Nussbaum was chief of the division of Genomic Medicine in the Department of Medicine. In August 2015 he became Chief Medical Officer of Invitae Corporation, a genetic information company.

24. Jeffrey Olgin, chief of the division of cardiology in the Department of Medicine. Interview, June 1, 2015.

25. Donna Ferriero, chair of the Department of Pediatrics, Interview March 3, 2015.

26. Talmadge King, Interview April 7, 2015. At the time of this interview, King was Chair of the Department of Medicine. In May 2015, he was appointed as Dean of the School of Medicine.

27. American Association of Medical Colleges, Report on Medical School Faculty salaries, 2013-2014. The AAMC provides online instructions on how to obtain a copy of this survey (Web 2 August 2015, at https://www.aamc.org/download/369956/data/currentgfanowissue.pdf).The authors examined the survey in the Academic Affairs division of the office of UCSF's Dean of the School of Medicine on July 14, 2015.

28. Kevin Shannon, Professor of Pediatrics, Division of Hematology/Oncology, Interview November 5, 2014.

29. UCSF Bridges Curriculum: Foundational Sciences. Web 24 August 2015, at http://meded.ucsf.edu/bridges/foundational-sciences .

30. Several types of disease have proved unusually amenable to genetic and molecular investigation: cancer, caused by mutations in oncogenes and tumor suppressor genes; infectious disease, where genomes of viruses and bacteria

furnished abundant therapeutic targets; disorders of the immune system (asthma, allergy, autoimmunity, and brain diseases like multiple sclerosis), in which developmental lineages of specialized cells opened avenues for unmasking pathogenesis and targets for treatment; neurology, where genetics and biochemistry are beginning to unravel epilepsy and neurodegenerative diseases. Research in other areas has made important advances: e.g., anti-cholesterol therapy for atherosclerosis, electrophysiologic technology for treating arrhythmias, micro-surgical technologies. Progress has been slower in a number of common and devastating diseases that may result from multiple mutations in myriad genes, such as diabetes, osteo-arthritis, and psychiatric disorders.

31. These roots began with a distinguished Epidemiology department, Steven Schroeder's founding of General Internal Medicine, a division of the Department of Medicine (1980), and Philip Lee's founding of the UCSF Institute for Health Policy Studies (1981; it is now the Philip R. Lee Institute for Health Policy Studies). As chair of the Department of Medicine from 1995 to 2006, Lee Goldman, an expert focused on delivery of health care, further expanded scholarship in this area.

32. Mike McCune. Telephone interview, March 9, 2015.

33. That is, approximately 65%, which was in addition to ~$6M in continuing support of clinical research centers (CRCs) for experimental study of patients. UCSF's CRCs had been supported for decades, and the 2006 grant added dollars for the CTSI to that continuing support.

34. For details, see UCSF Accelerate: Access CTSI services to enable research. Web 24 August 2015, at http://accelerate.ucsf.edu/training .

35. National Institutes of Health, Biomedical Research Workforce Working Group Report, June 14, 2012. Web 27 July 2015 at http://acd.od.nih.gov/biomedical_research_wgreport.pdf .

36. For UCSF's 13 matriculants in 2015, see UCSF Medical Scientist Training Program. Web 26 August 2015, at http://journals.lww.com/academicmedicine/pages/results.aspx?txtkeywords=Md-PhD+programs+meeting+their+goals .

37. LF Brass, et al. Are MD-PhD programs meeting their goals? An analysis of career choices made by graduates of 24 MD-PhD programs. Academic Medicine, 85:692-701, 2010.

38. Chiefs of three divisions in the Department of Medicine emphasized that both total salary and the K-award portion vary, depending on the division and the NIH institute, respectively. The numbers given here are guesstimates at best. In an email on September 1, 2015, Maye Chrisman, then Associate Chair for Finance and Administration in the Department of Medicine, wrote that the average K-awardee salary in her department (including 59 awardees

in every year of the award) was $160,000 per year (minimum $75,000, maximum $240,000), of which the average K-award itself pays $75,000-90,000. Thus our guesstimates of $80,000 from the K-award and $130,000 total are more or less in the right range for beginning awardees. A varying but substantial portion of the $50,000 difference between these two numbers, which is paid by departments, is earned by each awardees's clinical service.

39. Guerrero LR, Nakazono T, Davidson PL. NIH career development awards in Clinical and Translational Award Institutions; distinguishing characteristics of top performing sites. *Clin Transl Sci* 7:470-5, 2014. doi: 10.1111/cts.12187.

40. K Bibbins-Domingo and C. Razler. K-Awards in the Department of Medicine: 10 Year Analysis. Slide presentation (2014); communicated to the authors 5 February 2015.

41. Data derived from a personal communication, June 2, 2015, from Christine Ireland, plus several emails over the following week. Ms. Ireland is Deputy Director of the Clinical & Translational Science Training program within the CTSI at UCSF.

42. Perhaps, for instance, D is just a lonely person, G prone to detecting meaningless clues, and E too easily upset by imagined attitudes of colleagues. Worse, the interviewer's (unspoken but perhaps detectable) bias in favor of intensive scientific communication may have affected one or all of these interviews.

43. J. Grandis, Interview May 14, 2015. Associate Vice Chancellor of Clinical and Translational Research, Grandis came to UCSF in 2014.

Chapter 10

1. Holy Bible (King James Version). Genesis 41.

2. Depending on context, UCSF refers to "basic science" as comprising several distinct but overlapping subsets of faculty. The narrow definition of basic science departments (used in the context of proposal 2 in this chapter) combines eight departments whose (112 sponsored) faculty conduct primarily biological experiments. A broader definition combines those eight departments with four whose (85 sponsored) faculty conduct primarily social science research (e.g., in epidemiology and statistics, nursing, etc.). And sometimes this group of 197 faculty is included in an even broader group, which contains an additional 73 sponsored faculty in ORUs (see Table 8-2).

3. Such a committee might comprise chairs elected by each section and a rotating contingent of graduate program directors, plus two or three at-large members elected by BSD faculty.

4. About 95% of sponsored faculty in basic science departments of the School of

Medicine are in the ladder-rank series and thus would presumably be covered by the BSRF and any successor plan devised for the proposed BSD. Two less numerous groups of basic science faculty, however, would presumably not be covered by such a plan because (if they are primarily researchers) they obtain virtually all their salary from external sources; these include: i. a dozen or more adjunct faculty; ii. a tiny sprinkling of In Residence faculty.

5. The average rate of return on endowments is 5%. Division of $208M by 0.05 produces $4.16B.

6. Basic science faculty deserve part of this money because they already carry the burden of paying 50-70% of their salary from grants, and have no alternative source of funding except the university (chapter 8). While clinician-researchers can earn 25-30% of their salary from grants and still maintain a viable research program, they still must earn the remaining 70-75% from grants; if they cannot, they will be required to devote more than 25-30% time to clinical activity, further reducing their research productivity and prospects for external funding.

7. According to the Association of American Colleges' tabulation of PhD faculty salaries in basic science departments at UCSF in FY2014, 23% of School of Medicine faculty were associate professors, who received a median salary of $145,000. Let us assume the same median salary and percentage of associate professors for all 112 sponsored faculty in UCSF's basic science departments (including those in the dentistry and pharmacy schools, as well as medicine) in the same year. In that case, $75,000 per year for 23% of 112 faculty (26 individuals) would come to $1.95M—requiring, at a 5% payout, an endowment of $39M. That $1.95M payout could pay ~40% of salaries (including benefits, calculated as 29.7% of actual salary) for that same cohort of basic science associate professors. See the American Association of Medical Colleges, Report on Medical School Faculty salaries, 2013-2014; for more detail on this report, see chapter 8, reference *16*.

8. Email to all DOM faculty from Robert Wachter, Interim Chief of Medicine, December 18, 2015. (An author of this book received Wachter's email after the preceding main-text paragraph was written.) The DOM salary contributions will not be continued after promotion to the rank of Professor in Residence; individual associate professors who receive some salary dollars from the State Educational Appropriation (SEA) will receive only whatever IRAPS dollars are necessary to bring the total to $50,000 per year.

9. They may have assumed that UCSF's education of graduate students could not possibly be better than it is now. To the contrary, graduate programs could have been required to improve training as a condition for receiving payouts from the endowment. For instance, one of the authors has argued

that graduate education *can* be improved by reducing the time required to obtain a biomedical PhD degree (HR Bourne, Is 6 years too long to get a Ph.D. in biomedical science? *FASEB J* 29:357-360, 2015), and has suggested to his colleagues that UCSF is the right institution to meet the challenge.

10. N Ruiz-Bravo. Conversation with NIH: The Health of the Scientific Workforce. Presentation 4 December 2007. Web 29 November 2011. The Powerpoint version of this presentation can be found by initiating a search on the Office of Extramural Research's Public Websites Archive, at http://archives.nih.gov/asites/grants/05-29-2015/archive/ .

11. *S Rockey. More data on age and the workforce. NIH Office of Extramural Research, Extramural Nexus, March 15, 2015. Web 5 October 2015, at* http://nexus.od.nih.gov/all/2015/03/25/age-of-investigator/ .

12. A graduate program in the Watson School at Cold Spring Harbor makes PhDs faster. See Watson School. Cold Spring Harbor. Web November 12, 2014, at http://www.cshl.edu/images/stories/wsbs/ docs/WSBSstats. pdf . For description of an experiment to test whether other schools can match that example, see the paper cited in reference *9*, above.

13. For instance, shortening time-to-degree would reduce availability of cheap graduate-student labor in PIs' laboratories. The resulting labor shortage might be countered by replacing 2.5 graduate students with a well-trained PhD staff scientist—a move that could probably produce the same amount of effective labor but would require PIs to change organization of their labs, as others have recommended. See B Alberts, MW Kirschner, S Tilghman, and H Varmus, (2014) Rescuing US biomedical research from its systemic flaws. *Proc. Natl. Acad. Sci. USA* 111, 5773–5777. DOI: 10.1073/pnas. 1404402111

14. HR Bourne. *Paths to Innovation: Discovering recombinant DNA, oncogenes, and prions in one medical school, over one decade.* UC Medical Humanities Consortium and UC Press, 2011.

15. One such group might include, for example, an expert at constructing and analyzing "big data" in one silo, plus clinicians seeking to understand puzzling common clinical disorders (e.g., autism, asthma, epilepsy) in other silos. The group may have just discovered robust markers, biological and environmental, in subsets of patients suffering from such a disorder.

16. This paragraph's quotations are from the succinct, direct argument for UCSF's recent clinical expansion made by Robert Wachter, interim chair of UCSF's Department of Medicine. See: R. Wachter, UCSF Health: What it is and why it's important. UCSF Department of Medicine, Chair's Corner. December, 2015. Web 16 December 2015, at https://medicine.ucsf.edu/corner/ucsfhealth.html .

17. T. Cook. SFGH's Ward 86: Pioneering HIV/AIDS care for 30 years. UCSF

News Center, June 2011. Web 1 October 2015, at https://www.ucsf.edu/news/2011/06/9988/sfghs-ward-86-pioneering-hiv-aids-care-30-years .

18. RM Wachter and L Goldman, The emerging role of "hospitalists" in the American health care system. *New Engl J Med* 335:514-7, 1996.

Index

G

L

ladder-rank faculty at UCSF, 86–87, 97–98, 206n.4
Laret, Mark, 76, 179
local government contracts, as revenue source, 23
long-range development planning (LRDP)
asset leveraging and, 66
history of, 69–70
revenue source development and, 81–82
Lowenstein, Daniel, 122

M

managed care, impact on clinical services, 74–75
Martin, Joseph, 75
McCune, Mike, 150
medical research
contributions and discoveries at UCSF, 100–104
as essential requirement, 1
MD/PhD degrees and, 152–159
organizational structure of medical schools and, 99–104
sustainable funding model for, 1–6, 177–181
Mission Bay campus
capital funding for, 58–60, 192n.14
planning for, 70–71
modified total direct costs (MTDC)
calculation of, 40–41
Organized Research Units, 105–108
salaries and pensions for faculty and staff and, 51–53
Moritz, Michael, 31–32
Muddlement-Uncertainty Principle (M-UP)
indirect cost calculations and, 36–41
non-federal research grants and contracts, indirect cost recovery on, 45–48
research space costs and, 106–108, 197n.13
unrecovered indirect costs and, 52–53

N

National Institutes of Health (NIH)
advantages of funding from, 49–50
appropriations to, 194n.17
clinical research funding by, 141–148, 157–163
grants to UCSF clinical department, 108–111
indirect cost recovery rate for grants from, 43–45
negotiation costs, indirect cost recovery lost from, 44–45
"net" payout rates, for endowments and gifts, 29–31
non-endowment gifts, 27–31
non-sponsored salary sources, for UCSF faculty, 89–98

O

operating/capital leases
capital improvement funding and, 63–64
facilities funding and, 59–60
operating costs, buildings and facilities, 81–82
Operational Excellence (OE) program, 78
opportunity costs, capital improvements, 82
ordinary debt, facilities funding and, 59–60
organizational structure of UCSF
basic science department, 116–119
clinical research administration, 137–140, 142–148, 159–163
finances, culture and expansion of, 88–89
growth of clinical department and, 108–111
overview, 7–8, 99–104, 195n.8
quantitative comparisons of departmental research, 105–108
salaries and pensions for faculty, 83–89
silos in clinical research and, 175–177
sustainability of research and, 177–181
Organized Research (OR) costs
indirect cost calculations and, 38–41

Made in the USA
Columbia, SC
20 March 2020